Mayo Roots

Profiling the Origins of Mayo Clinic

ISBN 0-9627865-0-0

Mayo Roots

Profiling the Origins of Mayo Clinic

By

Clark W. Nelson

Mayo Historical Unit
Mayo Foundation

· Foreword ·

In the 1920s, Dr. William J. Mayo began a Clinic-wide effort to collect memorabilia relating to his father, Dr. William Worrall Mayo. He hoped that the material would have informational and inspirational value for future generations of Clinic people. Following the deaths of the Mayo brothers in 1939, individuals at the Clinic continued assembling Mayo memorabilia.

These initial efforts led to establishment of the first Mayo Historical Committee in 1952. Since then, many committees have devoted time to collecting, selecting, and preserving memorabilia. By appreciating the past, new generations can understand the ideals of service that guide Mayo's institutions as they evolve to meet challenges and opportunities of patient care in each decade.

This book is a compilation of articles that Clark Nelson, Mayo's historical archivist, authored for various Mayo Clinic periodicals. Articles first appeared in several internal newsletters, then in a "Mayo Vignettes" series published in *The Mayo Alumnus* magazine, and in a "Historical Profiles of Mayo" series carried by our monthly medical journal, *Mayo Clinic Proceedings*.

For easy access, the sketches are grouped into divisions and chapters whose titles reflect their content. Where available, photographs are included. This collection covers selected highlights of the Mayo enterprise and its beginnings in Rochester, Minnesota.

On behalf of the Mayo Historical Committee, I want to thank Clark Nelson for a job well done and recommend this informative and entertaining work.

> Mayo Historical Committee
> John R. Hodgson, M.D., Chairman

· Preface and Acknowledgments ·

The Mayo story spans more than 125 years of growth. Its roots are entwined in the American frontier movement that led to settlement of the Upper Midwest. Dr. William Worrall Mayo was an English immigrant who, like thousands of others, followed rivers and primitive roads west to reach rich soils waiting to be cultivated in America's heartland. Stirred by the freedom that his new homeland offered, and its potential for development, the elder Mayo sought to leave a legacy that would enrich those who followed.

After his two sons, Drs. William J. Mayo and Charles H. Mayo, joined his medical practice in Rochester in the 1880s, Saint Marys Hospital was opened by the Sisters of Saint Francis in 1889. The stage was then set for the development of America's pioneering private group practice of medicine. For the next 50 years, the Mayo brothers devoted the rest of their lives to developing and refining their integrated system of health care.

A high point occurred in 1919, when the Mayo brothers established Mayo Properties Association, today's Mayo Foundation. This not-for-profit organization became the vehicle that continues the Mayos' legacy of service today, and will do so for generations to come.

For those who wish a more detailed insight into Mayo and its formative years, *The Doctors Mayo* by Helen Clapesattle remains the definitive work. It is currently available through Mayo Foundation and many Rochester bookstores and newsstands.

It is perhaps indicative of what Dr. Will called "the spirit of the Clinic" that this work of historical reflection signals a new era in Mayo's technology. *Mayo Roots* is the institution's first book to be designed, edited, and typeset on an electronic desktop publishing system.

Publication of *Mayo Roots* is a classic example of the medical center's "team approach," and I am particularly appreciative of and indebted to the following colleagues:

MAYO HISTORICAL COMMITTEE: Dr. John R. Hodgson, chairman, whose steady support, and personal involvement with the preparation of the list of names, has made this publication possible.

Dale G. Chrysler, secretary, and Richard C. Spavin, past secretary, particularly Mr. Chrysler, who spent extra hours with administrative details and input.

MAYO MEDICAL VENTURES: David E. Swanson, whose seasoned eye has helped create and steer the work through the publication pathways. Matthew D. Dacy, whose sensitive copy editing and watchful hand has helped ensure a readable, well-produced volume. Joan L. Benjamin, who carefully prepared the final version of the manuscript in electronic form. Lindsay A.E. Shorter and Vicki M. Duffney, who have supplied administrative support in marketing and distribution.

MAYO VISUAL INFORMATION: (Medical Graphics) Marjorie G. Durhman, whose sensitivity to the written word and the supporting photos has produced a pleasing layout and design. (Photography) Sandra K. Gaspar, Elman A. Hanken, Mary C. Pederson, Merlin K. Schreiber, Karen M. Sprenger, who supplied a wide range of photographic support with promptness and efficiency.

MAYO SECRETARIAL SERVICES: Sara J. Schwantz, who prepared the initial electronic version of the manuscript.

MAYO PURCHASING: Stephen Q. Sponsel, whose support in paper selection, boxing, and printing has been vital.

MAYO HISTORICAL UNIT: Dacia Briese, who has been of immeasurable support in a variety of details.

MAYO PUBLICATIONS: Roberta J. Schwartz, Patricia J. Calvert, Jeanette Schlotthauer, and John L. Prickman, who provided advice and proofreading service.

SAINT MARYS HOSPITAL: Sister Lauren Weinandt, who has kindly shared photographs unavailable to us.

ROCHESTER METHODIST HOSPITAL: Sylvia A. Holt and Carol Ann Wallace, who also shared photos with us.

While gratefully acknowledging the many who have assisted, the author assumes responsibility for whatever inaccuracies may surface in the volume.

Clark W. Nelson

10

· TABLE OF CONTENTS ·

SECTION I — THE DRS. MAYO

SECTION II — ACTIVITIES AND HONORS OF THE DRS. MAYO

SECTION III — DEVELOPMENT OF MAYO CLINIC AND MAYO FOUNDATION

SECTION IV — MAYO OFFICE FACILITIES

SECTION V — MAYO HOSPITAL FACILITIES

SECTION VI — MEDICINE AND RESEARCH AT MAYO

SECTION VII — EDUCATION AT MAYO

SECTION VIII — MAYO ACCOMPLISHMENTS AND ACTIVITIES

· SECTION I ·

The Drs. Mayo

After Dr. William Worrall Mayo moved his growing family to Rochester in the 1860s, he developed a successful medical practice motivated by high ideals of service to his patients. When his sons, William James and Charles Horace, joined him in practice in the 1880s, they eagerly sought ways to improve the excellence of their father's patient care. Bolstered by the emergence of scientific medicine, Dr. Will and Dr. Charlie evolved in Rochester a unique blend of sensitive patient care delivered by a team of dedicated specialists who represent the best knowledge available in the science of medicine.

Dr. William Worrall Mayo's Arrival in Rochester

Dr. William Worrall Mayo arrived in Rochester, Minnesota, from nearby Le Sueur in 1863, when the war between the North and South was in progress. In 1861, Dr. Mayo had volunteered for duty in the Union forces. Because his application as regimental surgeon was denied, the "little doctor" began looking for other ways to serve the Northern cause.

When the federal conscription act was passed in 1863, Minnesota was divided into two districts with an enrollment board in each to select recruits. Dr. Mayo secured the examining surgeon position on the board that covered the southern half of the state. In May 1863, he reported for duty at the board's new headquarters in Rochester, Minnesota.

Dr. Mayo immediately liked the vitality of Rochester, with the railroad at its doorstep. By January 1864, he had bought property and moved his family from Le Sueur. It would be the last and most successful change of residence for the peripatetic founder of the famous medical family.

The elder Mayo was approximately 44 years old when he settled in Rochester. Almost 20 years had passed since his arrival in the United States from his home in Salford, England. During that time, William Worrall had followed the pattern of many Old Country emigrants. Not long after his ship docked in New York harbor, he began moving westward, settling for various periods in several communities in New York, Indiana, Missouri, and Minnesota. Along the way, he gathered experience as a pharmacist, a tailor, a physician and surgeon, a census taker, a farmer, a newspaper publisher, a justice of the peace, a ferryboat operator, and a veterinarian.

He also acquired a medical diploma and the conviction that physicians have a special calling filled with opportunity to help further the progress of their profession and communities. Dr. Mayo thrived on the challenges of the frontier and was often in the forefront of endeavors to improve community life.

Once settled in the city, Dr. Mayo developed a successful practice. His skills as a surgeon brought him area attention. As soon as his sons were able, they aided him in elementary ways. After they graduated from medical school in the 1880s, they joined him in "the Drs. Mayo" practice that culminated with the sons developing the Mayo group practice of medicine, which continues to flourish today.

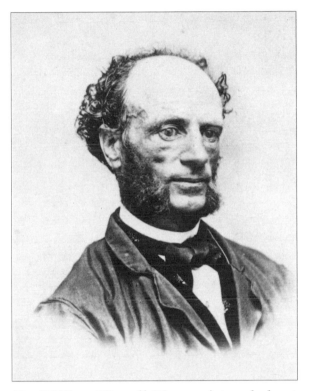

Dr. William Worrall Mayo, pictured about 1863. The founder of the famous medical family arrived in Rochester in 1863 as examiner of Civil War recruits. Around 44 years old, the "little doctor" had emigrated from England almost 20 years before and gradually moved west, stopping in New York, Indiana, Missouri, and finally Minnesota.

Early Medical Education of Dr. William Worrall Mayo

While residing in Lafayette, Indiana, in the late 1840s, William Worrall Mayo became a medical student of Dr. Elizur H. Deming, a prominent citizen and medical practitioner of the area.

Dr. Deming's education and professional involvement were beyond the norm for his time and location. He graduated with honors from Williams College in Massachusetts and later served as president of the Indiana Medical Association. When he became William Worrall's preceptor, he was a member of the faculty of the Indiana Medical College in La Porte. This school was among the pioneer efforts that served the medical needs of the growing population of frontier America.

Similar to most of the 38 medical schools in the United States during that period, the La Porte program required applicants to complete a three-year period of reading medical literature and assisting a practicing physician who acted as the student's preceptor. This preliminary training was the American version of the European apprentice system. Unfortunately, the requirements for licensing physicians in Indiana — and many other states — were so minimal that a would-be physician could bypass any portion — or all — of the recommended instruction and simply "hang out a shingle."

The elder Mayo was not of this bent. Apparently, the interest in science that he developed before leaving England led him to the preceptor arrangement with Dr. Deming, an association that culminated in William Worrall's enrollment at the Indiana Medical College. The dates that he attended the college are uncertain, however. Although he was later listed as a graduate of the school, there is no record of his matriculation. From the limited data available, he apparently attended the 1849-1850 session of the college, completed a thesis, passed his examination, and graduated on February 14, 1850. The school closed in 1850, and its building and records were destroyed by a fire in 1856.

Before closing, the Indiana Medical College at La Porte was a bright star among the area's medical schools. Its success caused nearby Rush Medical College in Chicago to propose a merger to eliminate the competition. In its final years, the college had an average annual enrollment of more than 100 students. Like many other schools, the college had neither an ambulatory clinic nor hospital facilities, although some surgical procedures were demonstrated in the school's amphitheaters. The school offered a course in pathology and physiology. It also boasted a microscope imported from England "at great expense." Interestingly, a microscope was not available to Harvard medical students until 1869.

Dr. Mayo became fascinated with microscopy and, during the course of his career, he purchased at least two microscopes. According to family tradition, he even mortgaged his home to purchase one of the instruments.

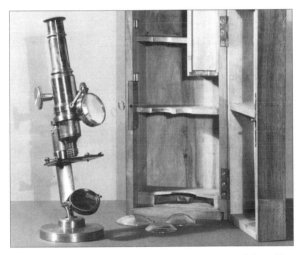

One of the early microscopes used by Dr. William Worrall Mayo. While attending Indiana Medical College, he became fascinated with the instrument's potential in medicine. In Minnesota, he was one of the few physicians to use a microscope regularly in practice.

While living in Indiana, William Worrall Mayo graduated from Indiana Medical College around 1850. In 1854, he received this M.D. degree from a forerunner of Washington University, St. Louis.

1862 Dakota (Sioux) War and Dr. W. W. Mayo

The Dakota uprising in western Minnesota occurred during the summer of 1862. The event is important to Mayo because of the role Dr. William Worrall Mayo played in taking care of the wounded during the outbreak. Violence between Native Americans and settlers in the upper Minnesota River valley began while the Civil War absorbed the political energies of the state. With the fall of Fort Sumter in April 1861, Minnesota became the first state to volunteer its services to the Union army.

Differences between the Dakota and their reservation agents came to a head during the middle of August 1862. For some time, the Dakota had been subjected to various schemes that made reservation life less than their treaties provided. The summer of 1862 was no different. When the Dakota gathered near Fort Ridgely to receive their annuity payments, the payments were once again delayed by the awkward and unfair tactics of bureaucrats in charge.

Their supplies low, the Dakota leaders decided to move. The outbreak that followed has generated an abundance of stories sprinkled with fact and fiction that even today are difficult to unravel. Once the Dakota took matters into their own hands, the agents and surrounding settlers fell victim to their attack. As relief forces mustered in Le Sueur and other surrounding communities, Dr. W. W. Mayo was among the physicians who came to aid survivors in the New Ulm area. For two weeks, these forces helped restore order and care for the wounded.

By December 1862, the offenders had been captured and tried. More than 300 Dakota were initially condemned to death. President Abraham Lincoln, however, delayed the executions, feeling them so unfair that he pardoned all but those convicted of rape and merciless murder. Thirty-eight were hanged in a mass execution in Mankato on the day after Christmas. Lincoln found the others guilty only of waging war, and these he pardoned.

Mother Mayo

On February 2, 1851, William Worrall Mayo married Louise Abigail Wright in Galene Woods, Michigan. Coming from upstate New York, with Scottish and English ancestry, Louise Mayo proved to be a steadfast partner for the elder Dr. Mayo in his varied career.

As mother of five surviving children (Gertrude Emily, Phoebe Louise, Sarah Frances, William James, and Charles Horace), the intelligent and industrious Mrs. Mayo provided a home life rich in common sense and purpose. She was a successful milliner who helped steady the family income in its early years. Her strong interest in astronomy and botany stimulated her children's appreciation of the sciences.

Mrs. Mayo became a skilled medical assistant to her husband, and in his absence aided patients until the doctor returned. Like Dr. Mayo, she lived a long, full life. She passed away July 15, 1915, during her 89th year.

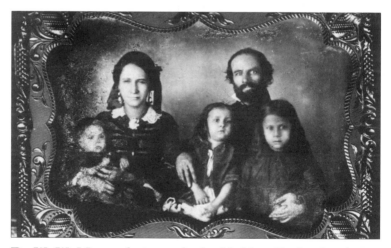

Dr. W. W. Mayo, photographed with his wife, Louise, in Le Sueur, Minnesota, around 1859. The children are Sarah, (left), Phoebe and Gertrude. Sarah died shortly after and William was born in 1861. Charles was born in Rochester in 1865.

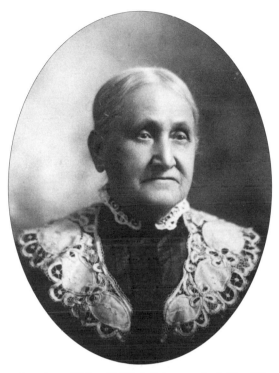

Louise Abigail Wright married Dr. W.
W. Mayo in 1851. As a milliner, she
steadied the early income of the family.
Her interest in science stimulated her
children's appreciation of that discipline.

Early Partners of the Elder Mayo

Before his two talented sons joined him, Dr. William Worrall Mayo held partnerships with several Rochester physicians.

In 1864, Dr. Mayo was associated with Dr. W. A. Hyde for about four months. The press described Dr. Hyde as a physician and surgeon who practiced in Rochester from 1863 to 1865.

Between 1867 and 1869, Dr. Mayo maintained partnership with Dr. Ole W. Anderson, a druggist and chemist. Dr. Mayo worked out of Dr. Anderson's drugstore. He also prepared and dispensed his own prescriptions there. Dr. Anderson was a respected member of Minnesota's medical profession. His *Norwegian Family Medicines* remained popular even after his death in 1920.

For a brief period around 1875, Dr. Seth Watkins Gould became a partner of the elder Dr. Mayo. He was a graduate of a Chicago eclectic medical school. In 1876, he left to practice in Mazeppa. In 1880, he returned to work with Dr. Mayo for a year before setting up practice in Pleasant Grove.

The last of Dr. Mayo's early partners was Dr. Elisha Wild Cross, the youngest of the popular Cross brothers. The Crosses were among the best-educated and most prominent physicians in pioneer Rochester. For about two years, 1876 to 1878, Drs. W. W. Mayo and E. W. Cross shared three rooms over Geisinger and Newton's drugstore on Broadway. The newspapers often carried notices of the major operations they performed together.

The Elder Mayo and his Rochester Colleagues

In addition to his early partners, Dr. W. W. Mayo enlisted the occasional services of other local physicians. Such arrangements often related to the performance of a surgical procedure. Among those who helped him were two women, Drs. Ida Clarke and Harriet E. Preston.

Dr. Clarke came to Rochester in 1881 to join Dr. Mary Jackson Whitney in the practice of obstetrics and diseases of women and children. About a year later, Dr. Whitney moved her practice to Minneapolis. Dr. Clarke remained in Rochester and became highly respected for her work. Born in Ohio in 1853, Dr. Clarke received the M.D. degree from the Woman's Medical College of Pennsylvania in 1878. After three years of practice in Lisbon, Ohio, she came to Rochester. Clarke was both a physician and a surgeon, and accounts of her surgical activities — including her assisting the elder Mayo and his son, Dr. William J. Mayo, in an ovariotomy and other procedures — were mentioned often in Rochester newspapers between 1881 and 1889. Dr. Clarke returned to Ohio to care for her widowed mother in 1889. She remained in active practice there until 1921.

Dr. Harriet E. Preston also assisted Dr. Mayo on occasion. An 1868 graduate of the Woman's Medical College of Pennsylvania, she practiced medicine and surgery in Rochester from 1869 to 1873, when she moved to St. Paul.

Her work was highly regarded by Dr. Mayo, and he acknowledged her assistance in various operations in a surgical report published in 1871. Her ability prompted him to request that she be admitted to the Minnesota State Medical Society in 1870. Her admission was refused, and for the next decade, Dr. Preston's candidacy for membership received no support. In 1880, the sentiments of the society's membership finally changed, and she became one of the first three women admitted to the medical society.

Dr. Will at Michigan University

When the elder Mayo began thinking about a medical school for William James, his eldest son, he was aware of the revolutionary changes taking place in American medical education. Dr. Mayo helped prepare a lengthy report on education for the state medical society that cited Harvard College as setting a new standard with a three-year graded course.

In 1880, the University of Michigan joined Harvard's lead and was among the first to introduce a similar three-year medical program. The university had also erected, some three years earlier, the "first real university hospital" in the country. Using the pavilion style of the Civil War, the frame facility had a 10-year life expectancy. At that time, such structures were burned after several years of use in an effort to fight infection. The work of Pasteur and Lister was yet to make a significant impact. Dr. Mayo thought that its hospital and longer curriculum made the University of Michigan a good choice for young Will, then 19 years of age. Will left for Michigan on September 16, 1880, on his first trip from home alone.

For the next three years, Will was, as he later recalled, thrilled and inspired. He became an underdemonstrator during his junior and senior years in Professor Corydon L. Ford's course in anatomy. During the long hours in the poorly ventilated dissecting rooms, he acquired a lifelong distaste for smoking. Despite this unpleasant distraction, Will developed a long-standing enthusiasm for anatomy.

Besides anatomy, he enjoyed the course in surgery offered by Donald Maclean. A devoted teacher, Professor Maclean chose Will to be an assistant in surgery during his senior year.

While at Michigan, Will also found time for boxing. He won the university championship in the 133-pound class. Other extracurricular activities included a founding membership of the social fraternity Nu Sigma Nu in 1882.

During Will's training at Michigan, Dr. Henry Sewall, the new professor of physiology, interviewed three of the best students to assess their learning. William Mayo, Franklin Mall, and Walter Courtney were chosen. After their interview, Dr. Sewall reported that all three of them would never succeed in medicine, either in theory or in practice. All three later became nationally prominent, and the Sewall story became a favorite among Michigan alumni.

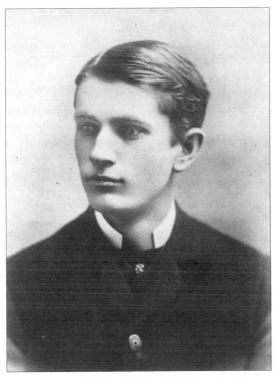

Graduation photo of Dr. William J. Mayo, taken for the University of Michigan in 1883. Dr. Will completed a three-year medical program there and found time to be a school boxing champion. Inspired in his studies, he looked forward to joining his father's Rochester practice.

In the spring of 1883, young William Mayo was about to graduate from the University of Michigan. He was almost 22 years old. In a letter to his older sister, Gertrude Berkman, on May 5, 1883, he revealed his enthusiasm and expectations for his future in medicine:

My dear sister Trude — This is the first time when I have had anything to write you, I have had time to do it. A member of our class died today, a very fine fellow and a good student — about a week ago he was bled from the arm — he thought he was too full of blood, the little cut in his arm suppurated and he had inflammation of the veins and died of blood poisoning. This makes 3 this year that have died out of our class and 2 have gone home to die of consumption. In our class of 120 in 3 years 12 men have died or broken down in their course and several in the class are injured in health, one in ten is a large proportion to give out. A good many do not learn easy — in fact should never have entered a profession. The course is hard, but some are peculiarly adapted to this kind of a life and I guess I am one of them as I have never been sick a day nor missed a meal and have worked right along and have a good time too. And when I get home some of the rest of us must have a good time — for we are really all one family.

Don't let Father work too hard — and when I get home I will give him more time to run the farm and rest, for I am anxious to get out and put my shoulder to the wheel for our common good.

For I am in love with my profession and with hard study and work with plenty of time, hope to make a success, but do not expect to do it in a day.

When Will's commencement came on June 28, 1883, Phoebe Mayo, another sister, made the trip from Rochester to represent the family. Following graduation, Dr. Will returned home to join his father in practice.

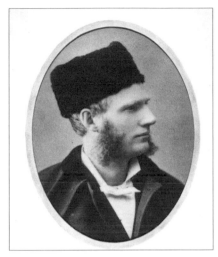

Dr. Donald Maclean was Will's professor of surgery at the University of Michigan. He chose Will to be an assistant in surgery during his senior year.

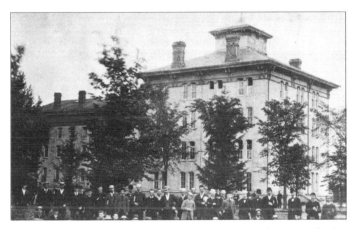

Dr. Will's class of 1883 posed in front of the University of Michigan's medical school building. Will was almost 22 years old at graduation on June 28, 1883.

Dr. Will's Marriage

The marriage of Dr. William J. Mayo and Hattie May Damon took place in the fall of 1884. During that time, Dr. Will was busily engaged in the growing medical practice of the Drs. Mayo in Rochester. It had been more than a year since he graduated from medical school at the University of Michigan and entered his father's practice. During 1884, Dr. Will traveled to New York City to complete some postgraduate medical training.

Upon his return, he married Hattie Damon, his best girl. As young children, they had attended school at the same time in Rochester. Hattie's father was a pioneer jeweler in the city who served as an alderman. Hattie was a graduate of Carleton College, Northfield, Minnesota.

The Mayo-Damon marriage took place on the evening of November 20, 1884, in the home of Hattie's parents at 427 Glencoe Street, now Sixth Avenue, Southwest. The original home was later remodeled and given as a wedding present by Dr. Will and Hattie to their daughter, Carrie, and her husband, Dr. Donald C. Balfour. Today it is part of the Civic League Day Nursery.

As reported in the local press, the "hymeneal" (wedding) started "promptly at seven" as the bridal pair took their places, and Rev. Bradshaw performed the ceremony "in his happiest style." Following the rites, dinner was served in the Damon dining room.

After their marriage, Dr. Will and Hattie bought an "elegant cherry bedroom set" and moved into their first home, the old Mayo family house on the site of the Siebens Building.

The couple celebrated their 50th wedding anniversary in 1934. Five children were born to them: Worrall, Helen, and William, who died in infancy; and Carrie and Phoebe, who later married Clinic physicians.

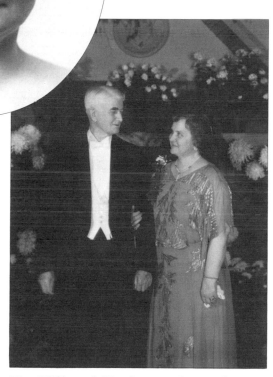

Hattie Damon married Dr. Will in 1884. They had been classmates while growing up in Rochester. She was a Carleton College graduate.

Dr. Will and Hattie posed together on their 50th wedding anniversary in 1934. Of their five children, two girls, Carrie and Phoebe, survived beyond infancy.

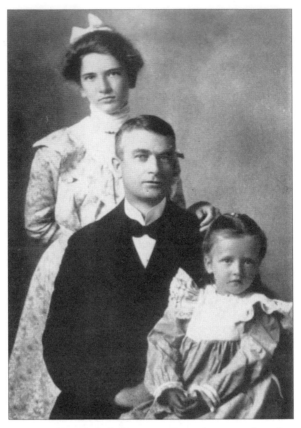

Dr. Will with his two daughters, Carrie (standing) and Phoebe. Both daughters later married Clinic surgeons. Carrie wed Dr. Donald C. Balfour, Sr., and Phoebe married Dr. Waltman Walters.

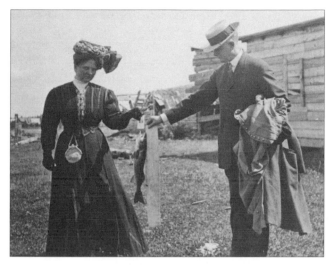

Dr. Will measures Hattie's "catch of the day." The Mayos enjoyed camping, boating, and fishing. The Mayo brothers built a cottage on the nearby lake at Oronoco where their families took turns enjoying short vacations.

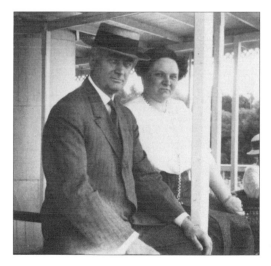

Dr. Will and Hattie were especially fond of relaxing on the Mississippi. When the automobile made access to the river easy, the Mayo brothers gave up their Oronoco retreat and purchased a riverboat on which to study, relax, and entertain family, visitors, and Clinic staff.

Dr. Charlie and Northwestern University

Charles Horace Mayo received his M.D. degree from Northwestern University on March 27, 1888. His proud father, Dr. William Worrall Mayo, attended the graduation exercises in Chicago. This event marked the successful completion of the medical program that the youngest Mayo had entered three years before.

Interestingly, a family council made the decision to send Charlie Mayo to Northwestern. The Chicago school was chosen because it provided a different viewpoint from the University of Michigan, where the older brother, William James, had graduated. In 1885, Northwestern's medical program centered in the pioneer Chicago Medical College. During this period, the college joined such leaders in medical education as Harvard and the University of Michigan by introducing a three-year graded program that offered clinical experience along with instruction in the emerging science of medicine. Besides its three-year curriculum, Northwestern possessed another attraction. The school was situated in the midst of a medical community with many clinical opportunities to observe and learn. The older brother had discovered these clinics during Chicago stop-overs on his way to Michigan. The stimulus of these varied clinics continued to attract the brothers to Chicago for years after their medical school days.

At Northwestern, Charlie's friends remembered him as an average student. They considered him rather quiet, but friendly. His indifference to dress was evident.

The medical students were graded on a one-to-10 scale. Charlie received his lowest grade of seven in surgery and perfect scores in dermatology and punctuality. In the lecture halls, he was careful to pick front-center seats with a good view.

While Charlie didn't excel in the formalities of classroom surgery, friends later recalled that he had a knack for searching out clinics in Chicago where he could observe the surgical greats of the city. His vivid descriptions of these visits revealed his early interest in the details of surgery.

After graduation, Dr. Charlie continued his involvement with Northwestern. He received the degrees of M.A. in 1904 and LL.D., Honoris causa, in 1921 from the university. In 1926, he was a principal speaker during the cornerstone-laying ceremonies for the first five buildings on Northwestern's new McKinlock campus. Dr. Charlie was elected a trustee of the university in 1932.

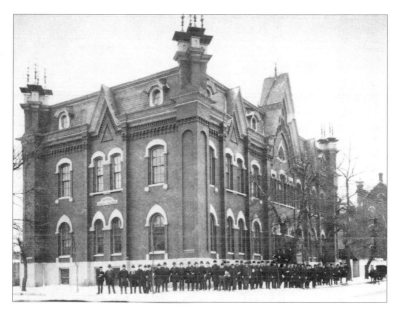

When Charlie attended the medical school of Northwestern University, its facilities included the pioneer Chicago Medical College (foreground) and Mercy Hospital (distance). The college had recently been absorbed by Northwestern.

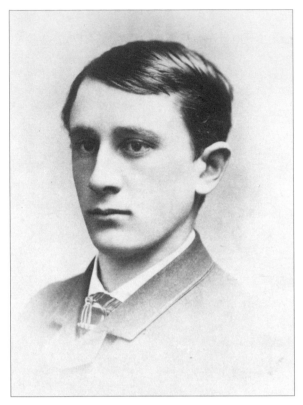

A family council made the decision that Charles H. Mayo would attend medical school at Northwestern. Charlie was a frequent visitor at surgical clinics in Chicago. He graduated from Northwestern in 1888 and maintained ties with the university throughout his life.

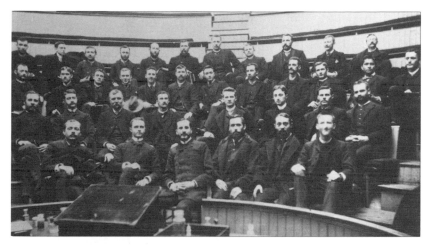

Dr. Charlie's graduation class of 1888 posed in the medical school of Northwestern University. Charlie is seated third from left in the third row.

Dr. Charlie's Marriage

When Saint Marys Hospital opened in the fall of 1889, young Edith Graham was put in temporary charge of its nursing staff. She was a Rochester native and a recent graduate of the school of nursing at Women's Hospital in Chicago. For the first few weeks, she assisted the Sisters of Saint Francis at the hospital, while informally instructing them on the requirements of nursing. After this brief interlude, she returned to her regular duties with the Mayo practice as anesthetist, office nurse, and general bookkeeper and secretary.

Edith Graham was a small, lively, attractive woman who was rejected on her first case in Chicago because the doctor thought her too beautiful to be a nurse. In Rochester, young Dr. Charlie found her equally attractive and on April 5, 1893, he married her.

The wedding ceremony was a simple one in the Graham home. Unfortunately, the happy event was marred by one small mishap. As the groom was hurrying out to the Graham home on foot, he tried leaping over a small stream and fell into it. The marriage ceremony was delayed while Dr. Charlie's clothes dried out.

The union of Dr. Charles H. Mayo and Edith Maria Graham was especially happy and successful. Because of her nursing background, she shared her husband's medical interests. On their wedding trip, they made rounds of several eastern medical centers.

Returning to Rochester, the newlyweds lived with Dr. Will and his wife, Hattie, in the home they had built on the site of today's College Apartments. Dr. Charlie and Edith soon built their "Red House" next door and began a family of eight children. In the 1910s, they built Mayowood and moved their growing family to the country.

After Dr. Charlie's death, Edith Graham Mayo became American Mother of the Year for 1940. Three years later, in 1943, she passed away. A bronze statue was erected to her memory in 1953 at Saint Marys Hospital. It is the work of her granddaughter, Mayo Kooiman.

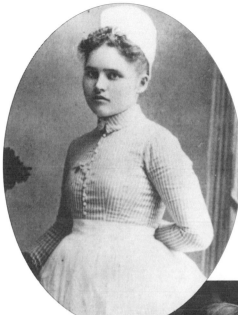

Edith Graham and her sister, Dinah, were the first trained nurses at Saint Marys Hospital. Educated in Chicago, Edith was rejected on her first case because the doctor thought her too beautiful to be a nurse. She married Dr. Charlie Mayo in 1893.

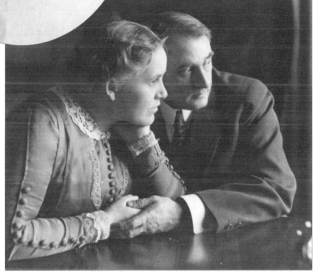

Edith Graham Mayo and Dr. Charlie, photographed around 1920. Of their eight children, two died in infancy. Edith became American Mother of the Year in 1940.

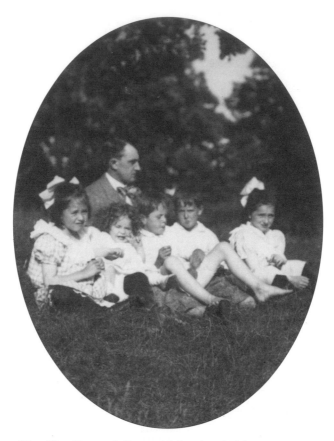

Dr. Charlie and five of his six children on the
lawn at Mayowood, his country estate. From
left: Dorothy, Louise, Charles William (later a
Mayo surgeon), Joseph Graham (later a Mayo
physician), and Edith.

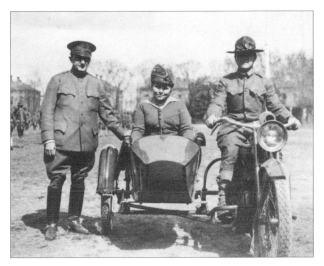

Dr. Charlie (left) with Edith on a visit to an eastern military camp during World War I. The Mayo brothers alternated duty in the office of the Surgeon General of the Army during the conflict.

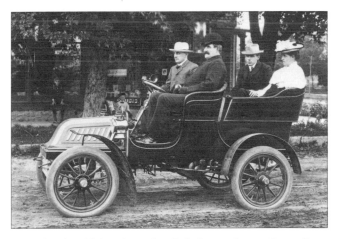

Dr. Charlie (driver) and Edith hosted two Canadian physicians in Rochester around 1910. Dr. Charlie purchased the first motorcar in Rochester.

Illness of Dr. Charlie

In the latter part of 1911, Dr. Charles H. Mayo was on his way home from a meeting of the Southern Surgical Association in Washington, D.C., when he suddenly became ill in New York City. Dr. Charlie diagnosed his difficulty as gallstones. The physicians who were called in, however, said it was appendicitis. Dr. Joseph Blake performed an operation to remove Dr. Charlie's appendix.

Dr. Will received news of his brother's illness in Rochester at 4 a.m., and within half an hour, he and Florence Henderson, Dr. Charlie's anesthetist, were speeding towards Winona on a locomotive engine, hoping to catch the morning train to Chicago. In the meantime, news of the emergency reached Winona, and by the time Dr. Will arrived, a special train was ready for the trip to Chicago. As soon as Dr. Will's party boarded, railroad personnel set out to break all records for an emergency trip, as the "special" sped past passenger and freight trains waiting on sidings. Arriving in Chicago, Dr. Will's party was able to catch the 18-hour flyer to New York City.

The newspapers had a field day with the story. Dramatic headlines appeared, describing almost mile by mile Dr. Will's dash to Dr. Charlie's bedside. Even the wild ride from the train to the hospital was reported — a ride that left Dr. Will wondering whether he could survive to see his brother.

The nation's press was quick to sense the public interest in Dr. Charlie's plight and carried stories of his illness in detail, followed by daily bulletins. Unfortunately, Dr. Charlie's health did not improve. He had a relapse, and another operation was scheduled for the removal of gallstones.

The story has a happy ending. Dr. Charlie's operation was a success and his convalescence uneventful. As before, the press covered the event with a variety of stories reporting on Dr. Charlie's progress and finally his return home to Rochester in January 1912.

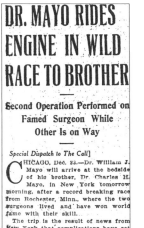

DR. MAYO RIDES ENGINE IN WILD RACE TO BROTHER

Second Operation Performed on Famed Surgeon While Other Is on Way

Special Dispatch to The Call]

CHICAGO, Dec. 23.—Dr. William J. Mayo will arrive at the bedside of his brother, Dr. Charles H. Mayo, in New York tomorrow morning, after a record breaking race from Rochester, Minn., where the two surgeons lived and have won world fame with their skill.

The trip is the result of news from New York that complications have set in following an operation on Dr.

Many accounts of the emergency appeared in the nation's press. This article from a San Francisco paper ran on December 24, 1911.

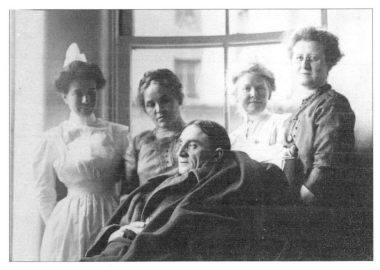

Dr. Charlie recovers from two emergency operations in a New York City hospital in 1911. Edith, his wife, is pictured at his side; his Rochester nurse, Florence Henderson, far right, stands with two unidentified New York nurses. The emergencies received national attention as Dr. Will rushed to his brother's bedside.

47

The Mayos and the Mississippi

Like many Minnesotans, the Mayo brothers had a fondness for the Mississippi River and its recreational potential. During their lifetimes, they owned three riverboats that became familiar sights on the Mississippi. Dr. Will was especially fond of the river and used the boats for relaxation and secluded study and writing. On occasion, he hosted Clinic staff and hospital employees on the vessels.

The first two Mayo boats, *Oronoco* and *Minnesota*, were steamers with paddle wheels. In 1906, the Mayo brothers bought an interest in *E. Rutledge*, later named *John H. Rich*, which had been built in 1881. The Mayos bought the boat outright in 1913 and changed its name to *Oronoco*. The vessel was 132.7 feet long by 30.5 feet wide. Its captain was Robert N. Cassidy of Winona.

In 1916, the Mayos had a new steamer built by the Howard Ship Yards Company of Jeffersonville, Indiana. They sold *Oronoco* that same year; the new owners renamed it *Ben Franklin*. The Mayos' new boat, *Minnesota*, was launched in September 1916. It featured a steel hull and was 130 feet long by 30 feet wide. In 1922, the Mayos sold *Minnesota* to the federal government, which renamed it *General Allen*.

That same year, the Mayos took possession of a new gas-engined, yacht-type riverboat called *North Star*. The new boat was 120 feet long and 21.8 feet wide. The former captain of *Minnesota*, John J. Richtman, was the chief officer. In 1938, the Mayos sold *North Star* to the Federal Barge Lines and gave the money to the Clinic's social service program.

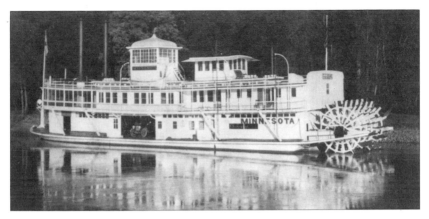

The *Minnesota* riverboat was built for the Mayo brothers, who used it between 1916 and 1922. The brothers were fond of the Mississippi River and its recreational opportunities. They used their first boat, *Oronoco*, from 1906 to 1916 and their last, *North Star*, from 1922 to 1938.

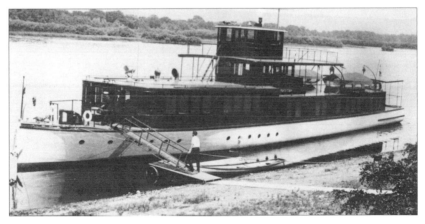

The Mayo brothers' last riverboat, *North Star*, was built in 1922. They sold the vessel in 1938 to the Federal Barge Lines and gave the money to the Clinic's social service section.

The Elder Mayo's Death

Dr. William Worrall Mayo died on March 6, 1911, only a few months before his 92nd birthday. He succumbed from complications of a farm accident a year earlier. At the time, Dr. Mayo attempted to free a stuck piece of farm machinery and, in the process, badly crushed his left hand and forearm.

Three operations became necessary, and the last resulted in amputation of the injured hand and forearm. The strain of this accident and its aftermath caused Dr. Mayo's health to fail rapidly and ultimately led to his passing. It was generally assumed that if not for this unfortunate occurrence, Dr. Mayo would have had several good years left. Up to that time, he had spent a life generally filled with vigor and good health.

Dr. Mayo's funeral took place the day after his death. Rochester's mayor ordered the city flags to be flown at half staff. City business was suspended during the simple service. At Dr. Mayo's request, the funeral was without eulogy and music. Rev. W. W. Fowler of the Episcopal Church officiated at the service in the Berkman residence (today, site of the Siebens Building). Before the service, many area residents came to the home for the reviewal.

Earlier that year, on February 4, 1911, William Worrall and Louise Abigail, his wife, had celebrated their 60th wedding anniversary. They were married on February 2, 1851, in Galene Woods, Michigan. At the time of their anniversary, they were the oldest married couple in Olmsted County.

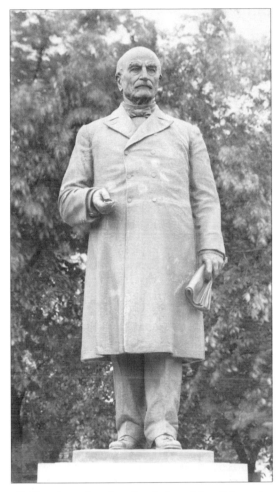

Following the death of the elder Mayo in 1911, a city-wide drive raised funds to erect a memorial statue. Leonard Crunelle of Chicago executed the bronze work, which was erected in Mayo Park in 1915. Today, the monument is prominently displayed before an entrance of the Mayo Civic Center.

Memorial Window for the Elder Mayo

The summer of 1929 was unique for the Mayo brothers. For the first time, they made a trip together to England. Previously it was customary for one of them to remain at the Clinic while the other was away.

The English trip was special for the brothers because it centered in Manchester. This area was their father's homeland, and the brothers felt that a meeting of the British Medical Association in Manchester presented a perfect opportunity for them to return. During their visit, the Mayo brothers received honorary Doctors of Law degrees from the University of Manchester.

Among the party traveling with them to Manchester was their eldest sister, Gertrude E. Berkman. She assisted in the Mayo family presentation of a memorial window to the Eccles Parish Church in memory of their father, Dr. William Worrall Mayo.

The elder Mayo was born in 1819 in the city of Salford in the ecclesiastical parish of Eccles. The memorial stained-glass window features five panels containing emblems and saints that typify his life, aspirations, and achievements.

The window contains depictions of: the coat of arms of Saint Christopher (patron saint of travelers), a symbol of Dr. Mayo's early pioneering life; Saint Joan of Arc and the Blessed Louise (Sister of Charity) as remembrances of the elder Mayo's wife, Louise, and her pioneering struggles; Saint George and his shield, representing the military and England; the arms of Saint Nicholas (patron of sailors), representing Dr. Mayo's coming to America; and Saint Francis of Assisi and the Blessed Virgin Mary, alluding to the founding of Saint Marys Hospital. The pelican (emblem of self-sacrifice) is in the bottom of the center panel as the root of all the other emblems. The window is the work of Francis H. Spear, a London artist.

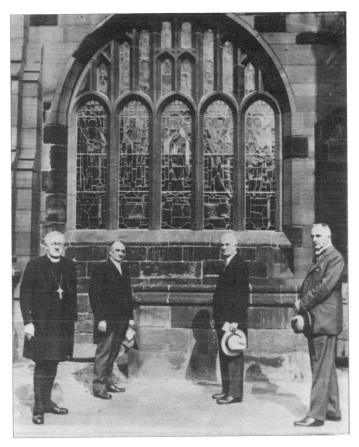

The Mayo brothers, center, before the stained-glass window that the family of Dr. W. W. Mayo gave to the Eccles Parish Church in Salford, England, his birthplace. Members of the family traveled to England for the dedication in 1929. The window features five panels displaying emblems and saints that typify the elder Mayo's life.

Dr. Will and Dr. Ochsner

The death of Dr. Albert J. Ochsner on July 26, 1925, brought forth tributes from physicians throughout America and abroad. Dr. William J. Mayo was particularly saddened by the passing of his close Chicago friend. Outside of the family circle, Dr. Will's friendship with Dr. Ochsner was probably the closest personal relationship that he ever had. Dr. Will characterized Dr. Ochsner as "my elder brother, guide, philosopher, and friend." The two men frequently visited medical centers together and shared their opinions and discoveries unselfishly.

Dr. Ochsner was born on April 3, 1858, in Baraboo, Wisconsin. He graduated from the University of Wisconsin in 1884 and received his M.D. degree from Rush Medical College in 1886. He practiced in Chicago from 1889 to 1925 and held a number of surgical professorships in that city. Prominent among these appointments was that of Chief Surgeon of Augustana Hospital, 1891 to 1925. He built Augustana from a small, 20-bed hospital to a 250-bed institution that attracted visiting physicians from abroad. He became particularly noted for his treatment of acute spreading peritonitis. Among his numerous professional activities, Dr. Ochsner was founder and president of the American College of Surgeons. He also received honors from professional associations at home and abroad.

Dr. Will wrote that Dr. Ochsner was a "man without vanity," and his death left him with a great personal loss that words could not express. Dr. Will further noted that, "Spiritually, morally, and professionally, I profited greatly by my association with him."

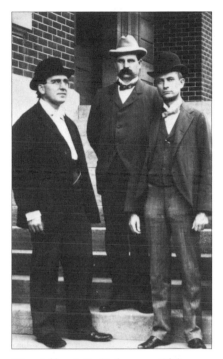

Dr. Albert J. Ochsner, Chicago, left, visiting with Dr. Will, right, and Dr. Arthur F. Kilbourne, superintendent of the Rochester State Hospital, around 1894. Ochsner was like an older brother to Dr. Will. The two often traveled together to medical gatherings and shared many pleasant hours with each other's family before Ochsner's death in 1925.

Dedication of Mayo Foundation House

On September 23, 1938, Dr. and Mrs. William J. Mayo gave their home to Mayo Foundation as a meeting place where people in medicine could exchange ideas for the "good of mankind." This gift fulfilled a dream that the Mayos had when they first planned the house around 1915.

Both Mayo brothers built large homes not long after the turn of the century. In that era, Rochester's facilities were limited, and it was difficult to house and entertain the many physicians who were flocking to visit Mayo's surgical clinics. Between 1910 and 1911, Dr. Charlie built a large home on his Mayowood farm in rural Rochester. Dr. Will followed by building a large home in Rochester between 1916 and 1918. The impressive new home contained 47 rooms arranged on two and one-half levels and had a five-story tower. Its design was reminiscent of an English manor house. (Dr. Will and his wife were of English descent.)

Franklin H. Ellerbe, founder of Ellerbe & Company of St. Paul, Minnesota, was the architect. He worked closely with Mrs. Mayo, who directed the building project for the family. Dr. Will made only one request — that a tower be included, similar to the one in his parents' home that his mother had used to pursue her hobby of astronomy.

The block on which the house was erected originally contained the pioneer brick home of Rochester's founder, George Head. At that time, the site was on the outskirts of the city, situated on a pleasant elevation overlooking Rochester.

Over the years, Mayo Foundation House has been a prominent facility in Mayo's educational programs. Even with decorative changes, many of the home's original features remain. Dr. Will's library with his personally graded series of books, the dining room, the living room, the organ, and the many family items scattered throughout the home still give it a personal look. In 1975, the home was included in the National Register of Historic Places.

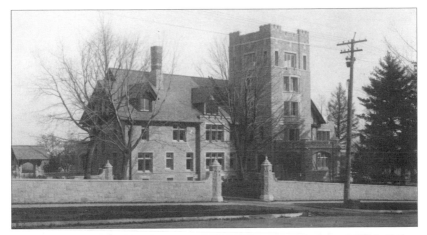

Mayo Foundation House was originally occupied in 1918 by the family of Dr. Will and Hattie. Designed by Ellerbe & Rounds, St. Paul, in close consultation with Hattie, the Mayo dwelling is like an English-style manor house. The tower is reminiscent of one Dr. Will's mother used in their farmhouse to view the stars. Dr. Will and Hattie gave the home to Mayo Foundation in 1938 as a meeting place where people in medicine could exchange ideas for the "good of mankind."

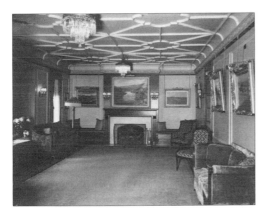

The living room of Mayo Foundation House, showing some early Mayo family furniture. The 47-room dwelling includes a dining room, library, organ, sleeping porch, Dr. Will's hideaway office, and a billiard room.

Mayowood

During the Minnesota summers, the state is full of activity as people enjoy the recreational and agricultural opportunities that the short season affords. The younger Mayo brother, Dr. Charlie, was an active participant in such summer pursuits. At his country home, Mayowood, he was an avid agriculturalist and conservationist. His concerns for the land and its wildlife anticipated the best of today's thinking.

Dr. Charlie devoted a goodly portion of his 3,000-acre estate to developing groves of trees and underbrush to help control erosion and provide space for recreation. He was a firm believer in some form of active recreation. He stressed the value of a good diet, rich in vitamins, coupled with plenty of exercise, preferably out of doors in the fresh air and sunshine.

As a flower lover, Dr. Charlie favored chrysanthemums, which he grew in his greenhouse at Mayowood. In 1934, he noted that he had 165 varieties of chrysanthemums growing along with other varieties of flowers.

He also was a strong supporter of the arts. Theater, music, dance, painting, and sculpture were all important to him. His only living daughter, Louise, is a talented sculptor and has produced artistic works on display at Mayo Clinic and in Dr. Charlie's home.

Mayowood was a game refuge where no shooting was permitted. The origins of Rochester's famous geese stems from when Dr. Charlie fed an earlier group of Canadian honkers on his country estate. Besides the geese, Dr. Charlie encouraged the growth of American and Japanese deer in the shelter of trees on his land. He also established a model dairy operation that helped set local standards for producing clean, pure milk.

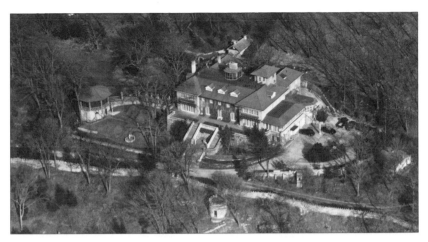

Dr. Charlie's home was erected on the Mayowood estate in 1910-1911. Dr. Charlie and Edith reared their children in the dwelling. It was the main house of the 3,000-acre estate on which Dr. Charlie developed a model dairy and practiced conservation of land and wildlife. In recent years, the home was given to the Olmsted County Historical Society.

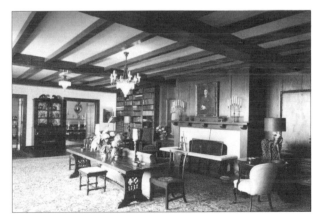

The largest room in the Big House at Mayowood is the long rectangular living room. Full-length portraits of Dr. Charlie's daughters-in-law hang on each side of the fireplace.

Damon House

The last Rochester home of Dr. and Mrs. William J. Mayo is located on the southwest corner of the block on which Mayo Foundation House stands. Now known as Damon House, the attractive two-and-one-half-story home was first occupied by the Mayo family in 1938. They built the dwelling to live in after they gave their larger home on the block to Mayo Foundation.

Today's use of the Damon name for this house stems from Hattie Damon, Dr. Will's wife. She had represented the family in designing and planning both homes on that property. Ellerbe & Company of St. Paul assisted her with architectural services in both endeavors.

Like Mayo Foundation House, Damon House is constructed of fireproof, reinforced concrete. Its exterior complements the larger home nearby and is finished with the same type of Kasota stone from quarries near Mankato, Minnesota. An attractive slate roof covers the dwelling.

The interior of the home is finished in the modern style of the 1930s. Extensive use of blond-finished wood paneling was one of its original features.

After Dr. Will died in 1939, Mrs. Mayo lived in the home until her death in 1952. Afterwards, Mayo Foundation acquired the property, and has used it for a variety of purposes over the years. Currently, institutional groups use the building for smaller gatherings.

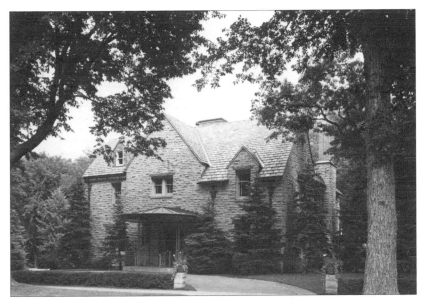

Dr. Will and Hattie moved into Damon House, their last Rochester home, in 1938. Hattie represented the family in planning the dwelling with Ellerbe & Co. Its exterior matched the larger home they had built on the block in 1918, but its interior reflects the styling of the 1930s.

Retirement of the Mayo Brothers

On July 1, 1928, Dr. William J. Mayo announced his decision to retire from the operating room. It was a difficult choice for the elder Mayo brother, then 67 years old. Dr. Will had previously spoken of retiring from surgery, but his colleagues persuaded him otherwise. After considerable thought, he decided that the role of surgical advisor would be the appropriate way to share his vast experience.

A year and a half later, Dr. Will's brother, Dr. Charles H. Mayo, discontinued his surgical activities. One morning in surgery, Dr. Charlie sustained a retinal hemorrhage. The irony was that it occurred the first day that his son, Dr. Charles W. Mayo, was to assist him. Despite complete rest, a series of strokes so reduced Dr. Charlie's capacity that he never operated again.

After they discontinued their surgical schedules, the Mayo brothers served the Clinic for many years. They frequently visited the Rochester hospitals and often observed in operating rooms. Their new freedom from surgical commitments also allowed them to travel together for the first time in years.

The Mayo brothers continued to serve on the Board of Governors of the Clinic until 1932. During the fall annual meeting of the Staff, Dr. Will announced that he and Dr. Charlie, along with Drs. William F. Braasch and Henry S. Plummer, would step down from the Board of Governors on December 31, 1932. At that time, the retirees formed an advisory committee available to the board. The brothers, however, never attended board meetings after 1932 or cast votes regarding the board's deliberations. With lifetime appointments, they did continue to serve until their deaths in 1939 on the Board of Members, governing body of Mayo Properties Association, forerunner of today's Mayo Foundation.

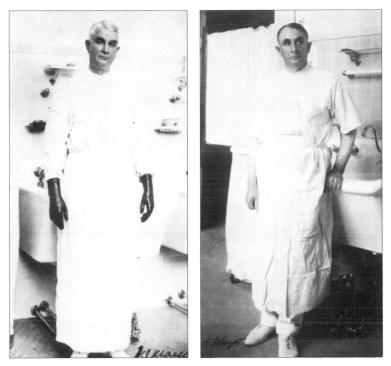

Dr. Will, left, and Dr. Charlie stand near scrub sinks at Saint Marys Hospital in the 1920s. Dr. Will stopped operating in 1928. After suffering a retinal hemorrhage, Dr. Charlie stopped a year and a half later. The brothers continued to serve the Clinic until their deaths in 1939.

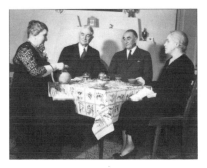

In their senior years, the Mayo brothers had more time to spend together with their families in Rochester and in their winter homes in Tucson, Arizona. This photograph is one of the last of Hattie and Dr. Will, left, and Dr. Charlie and Edith. It was taken in Arizona early in 1939, a few months before the brothers died.

Dr. Charlie's Death

Newspapers and radios across the United States announced the death of Dr. Charles H. Mayo on Friday, May 26, 1939, in Chicago. Dr. Charles W. Mayo announced that the death of his father, who was 73 years old, resulted from lobar pneumonia no. 3, a rare type that almost always was fatal.

Dr. Charlie became ill on May 18, during a visit to the Windy City. He was rushed to Mercy Hospital, where five physicians attended him, including two who came from Mayo. Despite their efforts, and lacking today's antibiotics, his strength continued to fail. During the next week, a blood transfusion from his son caused a brief rally, but Dr. Charlie soon slipped into semiconsciousness and then passed away that Friday afternoon. Family members were at his bedside. After his death, they arranged to accompany his body back to Rochester on the train.

Dr. Charlie's body lay in state in the lobby of the 1914 Mayo Clinic Building (today, site of the Siebens Building) from 11 a.m. to 5 p.m., on Sunday, May 28. The Clinic location gave more people an opportunity to pay their respects. The setting was also appropriate because the 1914 Building stood on the site of the original Mayo home, in which Dr. Charlie was born on July 19, 1865.

During the six-hour period, almost 10,000 people filed past Dr. Charlie's open casket, which was flanked by two honor guards from the American Legion post in Rochester. (Dr. Charlie had been a charter member of that post.) Afterward, the body was taken to Mayowood, Dr. Charlie's country home, where private services were held for family members and close friends the next afternoon.

Dr. Charlie's remains were then brought back to Rochester along a route that passed two landmarks in his life — Saint Marys Hospital, where he achieved international surgical fame, and the victorian-style frame home that he and his wife, Edith, built shortly after their marriage in 1893. As the hearse passed Saint Marys Hospital, white-uniformed nurses lined the street in tribute.

The cortege stopped at Calvary Episcopal Church, where a public service was held before an overflow crowd that included Gov. Harold Stassen of Minnesota. During the brief ritual, which was without eulogy, an additional 3,000 people stood outside the small church. Subsequently, the funeral procession proceeded to Oakwood Cemetery in east Rochester for brief graveside rites. Dr. Charlie's body was then buried in the Mayo family plot, where the remains of his parents and sister, along with those of two children of his own and three children of his elder brother, had been interred some years before.

Dr. Charlie's demise prompted expressions of sympathy and sorrow from hundreds of people in all walks of life and all areas of the world. As part of the local tribute, Mayo Clinic closed early and the Rochester business community suspended operations during the afternoon of his funeral.

Today, in reflecting on this unique co-founder of the Mayo enterprise, it is appropriate to recall a banquet given in Dr. Charlie's honor. The year was 1916; Dr. Charlie was newly elected as president of the American Medical Association.

On that occasion, Thomas Spillane, a Rochester attorney, said:

We who know him . . . know him for his charity and his love of the poor, and for his love for little children, and his interest in all that concerns them; his goodness to all, young and old . . . it is these things that get under the skin and make you feel that life is well worth living . . . that no matter how great may be his successes and his honors . . . he will always be to us gentle, kindly, Dr. Charlie.

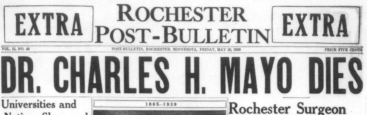

EXTRA | ROCHESTER POST-BULLETIN | EXTRA

VOL. 15, NO. 48   POST-BULLETIN, ROCHESTER, MINNESOTA, FRIDAY, MAY 26, 1939   PRICE FIVE CENTS

DR. CHARLES H. MAYO DIES

Universities and Nations Showered Honors on Mayo

Republic of France Conferred French Legion of Honor Upon Him—Awarded Distinguished Service Medal

From far-flung parts of the world honors were showered upon Dr. Charles H. Mayo during a life which belongs to history today.

Listing of awards, degrees, titles and active and honorary positions held by him would fill columns of space.

The honors were legion. The president of the country he loved so well came to Rochester in 1934 to pay tribute to him and his brother. Scholastic honors, degrees, awards and plaques were his by the score.

Among principal professional honors were his presidencies of the American Medical association in 1916 and the American College of Surgeons in 1924.

Foreigners Also Honored Surgeon

Great Britain, Ireland, Germany, France, Czechoslovakia, Yugoslavia, Italy, Spain, Mexico and Cuba honored him, and from his own country came the distinguished service medal awarded for his World war work. He was an officer of the French Legion of Honor and had the cross of the Royal Order of the Crown of Italy.

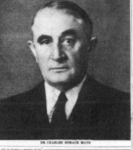

DR. CHARLES HORACE MAYO
1865—1939

'Dr. Charlie Stimulated Me By Example,' Brother Says

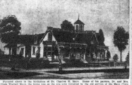

BIRTHPLACE OF DR. CHARLES H. MAYO

Rochester Surgeon Victim of Pneumonia In Chicago Hospital

Younger of Famous Brothers, 73 Years Old, Succumbs After 8-Day Illness --Native City and World Mourn Death

Dr. Charles H. Mayo died in Chicago at 4:55 p. m. today. Pneumonia claimed the world-famed 73-year-old surgeon, whose busy life ended in Mercy hospital after an illness of eight days.

Death came while members of his family were at his bedside, but absent was his older brother, Dr. William J. Mayo, who could not leave his home, where he is convalescing from a serious abdominal operation performed April 22.

The first of the brothers to die failed steadily during the day and the approach of death became clear when attending physicians indicated they believed a second blood transfusion would be futile.

"Dr. Mayo made an excellent fight, but the chances were against him from the start," said Dr. Walter McGuire, who explained that Dr. Mayo had type six and part of type three pneumonia, an unusual combination.

At the inception of the illness, Dr. Mayo's pulse was 102, with little cough and no fever, Dr. McGuire said.

Dr. Mayo was conscious only periodically throughout the day.

Early plans in Chicago were to bring the body to Rochester tomorrow morning.

Family at Bedside

Stricken in Chicago last Friday, he showed some improvement, but, weakened by previous illnesses and the passing years of a life that made his name known in distant lands, he began bowing to time's inevitable dictate when he suffered a relapse Wednesday night and his son, Dr. Charles W. Mayo, donated blood for a transfusion.

The son, the wife of the departed Dr. Charlie and three of his daughters, Mrs. Fred W. Rankin of Lexington, Ky., Mrs. John B. Hartzell of Detroit and Mrs. Louise Mayo Trenholm of Rochester, were with him when death came.

At the bedside, in addition to immediate members of the family were Mrs. Joseph Mayo, Dr. Herman J. Moersch, Dr. T. J. Dry of Rochester, Dr. R. S. Berghoff, medical director of the hospital, and Drs. Michael and Walter McGuire.

Although Dr. Mayo suffered periodical illness the past two years, his condition in recent months had been encouraging, and when he returned recently from Tucson, Ariz., where he spent the winter, he seemed improved generally.

Wanted to Return Here

Dr. Mayo would have returned to Rochester had attending physicians agreed. When he became ill for the last time he expressed desire to return here by airplane.

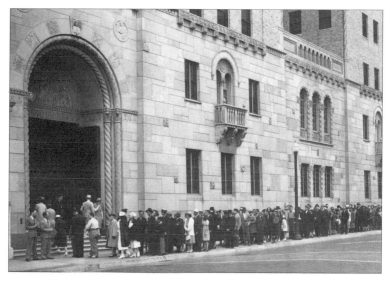

During a six-hour period, some 10,000 people filed past Dr. Charles H. Mayo's open casket on May 28, 1939. Dr. Charlie died in Chicago from pneumonia on May 26, and his body was returned to Rochester for burial.

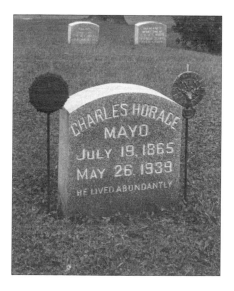

Dr. Will's Death

News media from across the nation solemnly announced that Dr. William J. Mayo died in his sleep during the early morning hours of Friday, July 28, 1939.

The passing of the 78-year-old co-founder of Mayo Clinic was the third somber event that staffs of the Clinic and Rochester hospitals had experienced that year. The first occurred on March 29, when Sister Mary Joseph Dempsey passed away. She was the pioneer superintendent of Saint Marys Hospital and a close associate of the Mayo brothers. The second loss took place on May 26, when Dr. Charles H. Mayo, the younger brother, died while on a trip to Chicago. When looking back to the opening days of 1939, there is little evidence that the Mayo brothers would not have continued to enjoy their senior years in fairly good health. Although Dr. Charlie had suffered some serious health problems a few years earlier, his condition had stabilized; in the late fall of 1938, the Mayo brothers and their wives journeyed to Tucson, Arizona, to spend the winter months in their adjoining cottages.

While in Tucson, Dr. Will took a short trip into Mexico. Upon his return, he began to experience gastrointestinal discomfort that failed to subside, prompting him to return to Rochester for a medical checkup. After his examination, Dr. Will underwent a stomach operation, which was performed by Dr. Waltman Walters, his son-in-law. Although the seriousness of his condition was recognized, Dr. Will rallied so encouragingly that Dr. Charlie, who had returned from Arizona to be with him, decided to make a previously planned trip to Chicago.

However, Dr. Charlie became ill with pneumonia while in Chicago and died. By the time Dr. Charlie's body was returned to Rochester, Dr. Will was too ill to attend his funeral. Dr. Will then underwent another operation, which was performed in his home and confirmed the critical nature of his gastric malignant lesion. Dr. Will's death soon followed, with his wife, his two daughters and their husbands, and Harry J. Harwick at his bedside.

Arrangements were made for Dr. Will's body to lie in state the following Sunday, July 30, at Mayo Foundation House, the home that he and his wife, Hattie, gave to Mayo Clinic in 1938. The hours for reviewal were 9 a.m. to 1 p.m. for the public and 1 p.m. to 3 p.m. for members of the Mayo staff. While the pipe organ in the home was softly played with favorite melodies of Dr. Will, some 6,000 people, along with scores of Mayo staff members, moved by the bier, which stood at the foot of the main stairway. Minnesota's Gov. Harold E. Stassen was among the early arrivals who came to pay respects.

Dr. Will's funeral service was held in the home at 4 p.m., with attendance by invitation only. A short service was conducted by the minister of the local Congregational Church, who was assisted by the rector of Calvary Episcopal Church. As part of the eulogy, Rev. George P. Sheridan said of Dr. Will: "He saw the trees before they appeared, the tomorrow before the sun rose, and dared to bring the future into the present."

The funeral procession then traveled through downtown Rochester past the closed doors of Mayo Clinic, as uniformed nurses from Saint Marys Hospital stood lining the street. As the cortege turned toward the cemetery, it passed another line of nurses standing beside Colonial Hospital, an affiliate of Mayo Clinic.

At Oakwood Cemetery, brief graveside rites were held and taps were sounded, before the remains of Dr. Will were placed in the family plot. After Dr. Will's burial, cards and letters continued to arrive in Rochester from throughout the world. To some, the passing of the Mayo brothers within two months of each other seemed a fitting, almost natural, ending for the two physicians who had worked so harmoniously together in establishing and developing the Mayo enterprise.

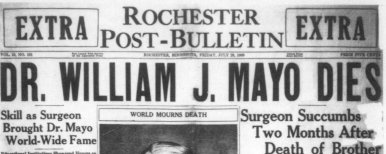

Rochester Post-Bulletin, July 28, 1939.

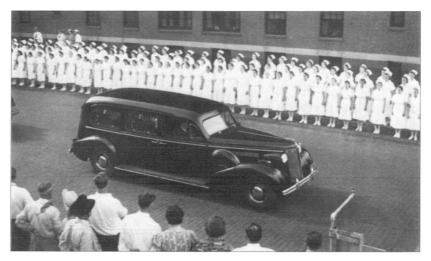

On the way to Oakwood Cemetery, Dr. Will's hearse passed a line of nurses standing alongside Colonial Hospital, a Mayo affiliate, on July 30, 1939. Dr. Will died in Rochester on July 28, 1939, from a stomach malignancy.

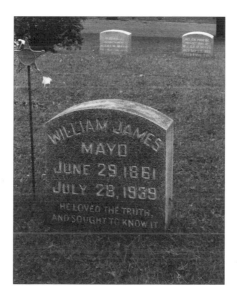

Dr. Will on Religion

An article on science and religion was sent to Dr. William J. Mayo in 1931. In response, he wrote:

The glory of medicine is that it is constantly moving forward, that there is always more to learn. The ills of today do not cloud the horizon of tomorrow, but act as a spur to greater effort. The triumph of the medical profession lies in the victory over physical ailments of man. The failure lies in an ability to appreciate and deal intelligently with the emotional instabilities of those physically ill or those with inherited or acquired instabilities of the nervous system which lead to miseries as grievous as though they were dependent on tangible physical causes. We must not forget that happiness is a state of mind, not necessarily of body, and that life is what each person believes it to be. The sick man needs faith, faith in his physician, but there comes a time when faith in a higher power may be necessary to sustain his morale. Notwithstanding the narrow creeds and misuse of authority which has so frequently characterized the church, religion based on the Sermon on the Mount and carrying the comfort of the Twenty-third Psalm of David, gives great assurance, no matter what the truth may be.

Mayo Genealogy

The following simplified chart identifies the early family members carrying the Mayo name and those Mayos who have become physicians.

William Worrall Mayo, M.D.   1819-1911

Louise Abigail Wright   1825-1915 (married 1851)
  —Horace Mayo (died at age six weeks)

    —Gertrude Emily Mayo   1853-1938

    —Phoebe Louise Mayo   1856-1885

    —Sarah Frances Mayo   1859-1860

—William James Mayo, M.D. 1861-1939

    Hattie May Damon   1864-1952 (married 1884)
      —Carrie Louise Mayo   1887-1960 (married Donald
                                       C. Balfour, M.D., deceased
                                       Mayo Staff)

      —Worrall Mayo   1889-1889

      —Helen Phoebe Mayo   1892-1893

      —William Damon Mayo   1893-1894

      —Phoebe Gertrude Mayo   1897-   (married Waltman
                                       Walters, M.D., deceased
                                       Mayo Staff)

—Charles Horace Mayo, M.D.   1865-1939

    Edith Maria Graham   1867-1943 (married 1893)
    —Margaret Mayo   1895-1895

    —Dorothy Mayo   1897-1960

    —Charles William Mayo, M.D.   1898-1968 (deceased Mayo
                                       Staff)
      Alyse (Alice) Varney Plank   1907-1967 (married 1927)
      —Mildred (Muff) Mayo
      —Charles Horace Mayo II, M.D. (former Mayo resident)

—Edward Martin (Ned) Mayo
—Joseph Graham Mayo (II)
   Joanne Ward (married 1951)
   —Joseph Graham Mayo III, M.D. (former Mayo resident)
   —Chester W. Mayo, M.D. (currently Mayo resident)
   —Edith Maria Mayo
—Alexander Steward Mayo

—Edith Mayo	1901-1982 (married Fred W. Rankin, M.D., deceased Mayo Staff)
—Joseph Graham Mayo, M.D.	1902-1936 (deceased Mayo Staff)
—Louise Mayo	1906-
—Rachel Mayo	1908-1910
—Esther Mayo	1909-1971 (married John B. Hartzell, M.D., deceased Mayo resident)

—Marilyn Mayo (adopted daughter) and John H. Nelson (foster son)

· SECTION II ·

Activities and Honors of the Drs. Mayo

The Mayos were active in developing their profession and community. Following their father's example, the Mayo brothers became leaders in professional associations and in city, state, and federal activities. Their contributions were acknowledged by a series of honors and memorials.

The Drs. Mayo and Organized Medicine

Throughout their careers, the Mayo brothers played leading roles in the development of organized medical practice in the United States.

Their awareness of the responsibility that physicians have to their profession was fostered early in their lives by their father, Dr. William Worrall Mayo. He was a staunch supporter of professional associations dedicated to improving the standards of medical practice.

In addition to his active membership in the American Medical Association (AMA), the senior Mayo was a founder of and officer in several state and local medical organizations. He helped reactivate the Minnesota State Medical Society after the Civil War and served as its president in 1872-1873. During his inaugural speech, he noted that the society's membership had become ". . . a grand brotherhood of science — who, in line of their duty, knows neither race or color when humanity is suffering, not even reserving to yourselves the right to avoid either danger or death by contagion or infection . . ."

Joining their father's medical practice in the 1880s, the Mayo brothers also became active members of various medical societies. In time, they were appointed to positions of responsibility at the local and state levels. First, Dr. William J. Mayo, the older brother, became president of the Minnesota State Medical Association in 1893-1894. Ten years later, at age 44, he became one of the youngest physicians to be elected president of the AMA (1905-1906).

In his presidential address, Dr. Will focused on the issues that confronted the medical profession of his day. He called for an enlightenment of the public by physicians to counteract commercial forces and their patented compounds. He decried the availability of such poisonous and intoxicating concoctions as "Kopp's Baby's Friend" and "Mother Winslow's Soothing Syrup," both of which contained opium. Dr. Will also spoke against fee splitting and other professional evils. He concluded with remarks on the need for continuing medical education as a means of furthering medical progress.

After serving in this post of national leadership, Dr. Will continued to participate in and lead many other national professional associations. Among those that he served as president were the Society of Clinical Surgeons (1911-1912), the American Surgical Association (1913-1914), and the American College of Surgeons (1918-1920).

Following in his father's and brother's footsteps, Dr. Charles H. Mayo, the younger brother, also became active in the various medical societies. He served as president of the Minnesota State Medical Association in 1905-1906. Subsequently, Dr. Charlie provided presidential leadership in numerous other associations, including the Western Surgical Association (1904-1905), the Society of Clinical Surgeons (1911-1912), the AMA (1916-1917), the American College of Surgeons (1924-1925), and the American Surgical Association (1931-1932).

Because Dr. Charlie's presidency of the AMA occurred during World War I, his presidential address dealt primarily with the war's influence on medicine, including commentaries on patriotism, education, and public health issues, in which he noted that ". . . the citizen is best made when a child."

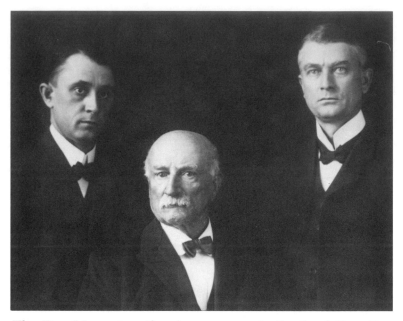

The Drs. Mayo, together in a rare portrait: the father, Dr. William Worrall Mayo, seated, and his sons, Dr. Charles H. Mayo, left, and Dr. William J. Mayo, standing. Active in Minnesota medical associations, the elder Mayo stimulated his sons, who subsequently played leading roles in the development of organized medicine in America.

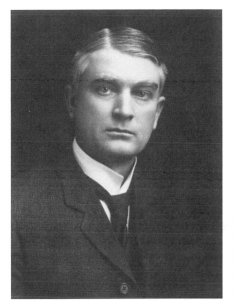

Dr. Will's photograph taken for his presidency of the American Medical Association in 1905-1906. He was the group's second-youngest president up to that time.

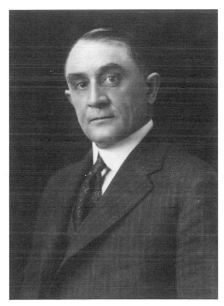

Dr. Charlie's photograph for his American Medical Association presidency in 1916-1917. As the group's leader during World War I, he urged support of the war effort.

Drs. Mayo and Community Service

Community service was a significant characteristic of the Mayos. The father, Dr. William Worrall Mayo, served his city in a number of capacities. He was a founder of the Rochester Public Library in 1865. He served as a member of the Rochester Board of Education from 1867 to 1870 and 1883 to 1889. In the fall of 1869, he was elected county coroner.

The elder Mayo was also instrumental in organizing the Rochester Board of Trade in 1881. He served as mayor of Rochester, 1882 to 1883, and alderman from his ward, 1885 to 1889. He was originally a member of the Republican Party, but joined the Democrats in 1870 to support the anti-monopoly and free-trade platform. The Farmers Alliance-Democratic ticket elected him state senator in 1890.

In 1865, the senior Mayo became a member of the city board of health. For several decades, he was intermittently active as chairman, secretary, or member of the board.

Dr. Mayo's famous sons also had a variety of public service experiences. Beginning in 1907, Dr. Will served for many years as a member of the Board of Regents, University of Minnesota. Dr. Charlie became health officer of Rochester in 1912. He held this post for many years and helped to foster many improvements in the health of the community. Like his father, Dr. Charlie served on the Rochester school board. He was influential in replacing wooden school buildings with fireproof structures. He promoted the establishment of the Rochester Community College in 1915, the first junior college in Minnesota. Along with his brother, Dr. Charlie presented funds to the school board for a number of years to employ a music director in the city schools.

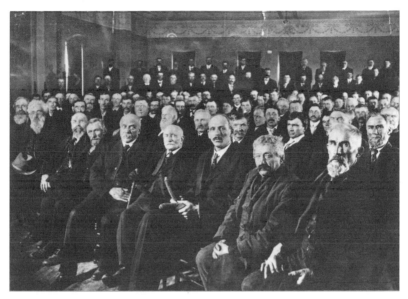

Dr. William Worrall Mayo at a Rochester area citizens' meeting around the 1890s. The elder Mayo was an example to his sons, who became active in community projects. W.W. Mayo is seated front row, fourth from right.

Early Rochester Education

After his arrival in Rochester in 1863, Dr. William Worrall Mayo became involved in many civic activities. One of the first was the Rochester Board of Education. Dr. Mayo was elected a member of the school board for the 1867-1870 term. He joined the board as its membership was planning a building for the city's education program. Beginning in 1855, the city housed its school in a log cabin, relocated it to several other makeshift structures and ended up with classes scattered throughout the courthouse. A year before Dr. Mayo joined the board, the city voted a tax of $25,000 to build a new schoolhouse. Construction of the new structure began the year that Dr. Mayo came on the board.

Central School was completed in 1868. It was then the tallest building in the city and cost about $75,000, including the land. The impressive structure stood on the block where the Mayo Building is today.

Dr. Mayo took his educational responsibilities seriously. While participating in an annual visit to the classrooms, he noted a number of defects in the educational programs. In his committee's report, he summarized:

. . . there was an apparent restlessness, an apathetic indifference to the higher achievements of the schoolroom, which showed us that some of the stronger wills before us had not yet been convinced that they were trifling with their own best interests.

It would seem from the action of some of these children as if they thought our City Fathers had . . . erected, at great expense, a gigantic playhouse for very large children with small ambitions; instead of a schoolhouse for instruction.

After leaving the board in 1870, Dr. Mayo was elected again in 1883. He served two more terms until 1889. His enthusiasm for educational opportunities never left him. When Hamline University was looking for a new home outside Red Wing, he was among the community leaders attempting to attract it to Rochester.

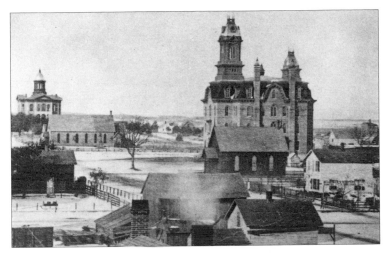

The imposing Central School, at the time of its construction in 1868. Dr. William Worrall Mayo was then active on the Rochester School Board. He later supported attempts to bring Hamline University to the city.

Rochester Parks

During the pleasant days of summer, many Rochester people enjoy the varied facilities in the city's attractive parks. The Mayo family and the Clinic were among the early supporters of such recreational areas in Rochester. During his term as mayor in 1882-83, Dr. William Worrall Mayo enthusiastically promoted establishment of a park near the present site of Mayo Park.

In January 1907, the Mayo brothers contributed money and land east of downtown Rochester for park purposes. The gift formed the major portion of today's Mayo Park. In 1909, an additional gift of land by the Mayos brought the total area of Mayo Park to 38 acres.

In 1908, the Mayo brothers also purchased and gave to the city four and one-half acres of land overlooking the city and Saint Marys Hospital. This observatory park in southwest Rochester is called Saint Marys Park.

In 1910, the Mayo brothers presented nine and one-half acres of property northeast of Mayo Park to the city for athletic use. Since then, Mayo Field has been the scene of many ball games.

Each of these parks contains a bronze tablet attached to a large boulder acknowledging the Mayo gift. The markers were placed there by the city in 1928. The bronze plaques are the work of Minneapolis sculptor Charles S. Wells.

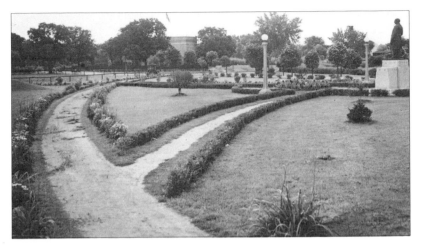

Mayo Park began with a gift of land and money from the Mayo brothers in 1909. Their father had long urged the development of parks. The brothers also gave land for the development of Saint Marys Park.

Good Roads and the Mayo Brothers

Shortly after the turn of the century and with the advent of the automobile, travel possibilities became greatly expanded. At first, the lack of well-drained gravel roads hindered all-season use of the motor car in many parts of the country. In the Upper Midwest, "good roads" became a popular theme for taxpayer groups that formed to address local conditions.

Dr. William J. Mayo, along with his brother, headed or participated in the efforts of such citizen organizations. In 1915, Dr. Will headed the Taxpayers' Good Roads Association of Olmsted County. The grass-roots association helped promote grading and graveling of county roads. As association leader, Dr. Will urged the construction of weatherproof roads "fit for the farmers to use every day, rain or shine."

The volunteer association held gatherings that often attracted large, enthusiastic audiences. On several occasions, the crowds numbered in the hundreds, with 400 being the highest counted. Their proceedings resembled political rallies, with musical entertainment included.

The activities of the Olmsted County group led to improved roads for the county. Various Clinic people and other community leaders often contributed funds, while local farmers provided time and labor for road construction. Road-building "bees" were popular and various sections of county thoroughfares were thereby improved.

Following these early efforts, the Mayo brothers also helped other concerned groups promote the paving and further upgrading of area and interstate roads. Dr. Will felt that better roads would help the citizens of crowded cities travel into the country, where they could better appreciate America.

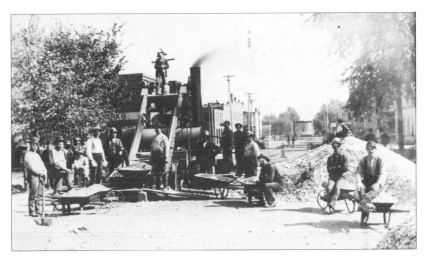

A road construction crew in Rochester around 1915. The Mayo brothers helped lead the movement to bring good roads to southeastern Minnesota.

Dr. Charlie and Public Health

The recycling of garbage is not new in Rochester. In 1916, Dr. Charles H. Mayo, acting in his capacity as Rochester's health officer, secured permission from the city council to control the collection and disposal of garbage. As part of his plan for processing the refuse, Dr. Charlie rented 30 acres of sandy land where he set up a feeding farm for purebred hogs. (This farm was adjacent to the site of the present Longfellow Elementary School on Marion Road, Southeast.) Here he had edible garbage fed to the hogs. In time, the fattened animals were sold and young ones purchased.

By 1920, the scheme had proven feasible, and Dr. Charlie presented the hog farm, complete with 400 hogs, to the city with the proviso that its income subsidize city health programs. For many years, the operation remained cost-effective, and in its early years even paid surpluses to the city. The activity continued until 1954. In that year, a new state law required cooking garbage before feeding it to the hogs. No economical means were available to accomplish this, and the farm operation disbanded.

The recycling activity was one of a number that Dr. Charlie introduced during his 25 years as Rochester's health officer. He was drafted to the post in 1912 by an aroused citizenry during a scarlet fever epidemic. During the outbreak, a delegation awakened Dr. Charlie one night at his home. They insisted that he immediately accept the health officer position. While still clad in his nightshirt and dressing gown, he became the new city health official.

Until his resignation in 1937, Dr. Charlie placed Rochester in the forefront of the public health movement in the Upper Midwest. He promoted scientific methods to control the spread of disease. He established a model dairy at Mayowood and successfully won the local battle to require pasteurization of milk.

Dr. Charlie persuaded the Olmsted County Medical Society to help sponsor weekly public health lectures. Other features of his innovative health program for the city included preschool and prenatal clinics, public school dental health clinics, and home nursing instruction. For some years, the Mayo brothers paid for any deficits that these programs incurred.

In recognition of these contributions, a new public health center was dedicated to the memory of Dr. Charles H. Mayo in 1950.

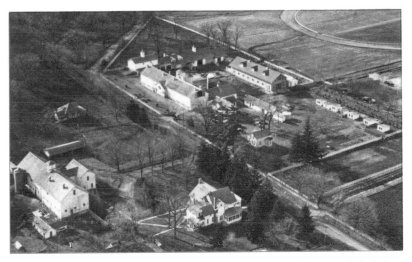

As Rochester's health officer, Dr. Charlie used his model dairy at Mayowood to promote the production of safe, clean milk. He was drafted as health officer in 1912. Before his resignation in 1937, Dr. Charlie placed Rochester among the area's public health leaders.

Mayo Brothers in the Army

When the United States declared war against Germany on April 6, 1917, many of the country's men expected to see overseas military service. The Mayo brothers were no exception. Some years before, they had enlisted in the reserves and had been commissioned first lieutenants in the Medical Reserve Corps. Dr. Will was appointed on November 21, 1912, and Dr. Charlie on January 16, 1913. Despite their expectations, neither of the Mayos served in France during World War I.

Instead, both Mayos initially served on the General Medical Board of the United States Council for National Defense shortly after it was formed in 1916 to prepare America for possible military action. After the declaration of war, Dr. William C. Gorgas, Surgeon General of the U.S. Army, asked Dr. Will to be a surgical consultant to his office in the nation's capital. Under Dr. Will's direction, a team of surgical experts was formed, which included both Mayo brothers. They alternated their military duty in the Surgeon General's office. In this fashion, the Mayo brothers were able to serve their country. Unfortunately, the heavy demands of the wartime years on their time and energy led to ill health in both men.

While on one of his Washington trips, Dr. Charlie contracted pneumonia, and Dr. Will came down with a severe case of jaundice that kept him away from the Clinic for two months. This was the first time either of the brothers had been away from the Clinic for an extended period.

In 1921, they were both commissioned brigadier generals in the Medical Reserve Corps of the U.S. Army. In March 1926, the Mayo brothers were honored for their wartime efforts with the Distinguished Service Medal of the United States.

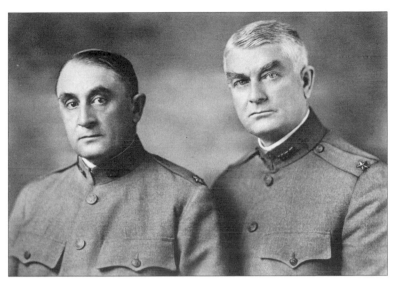

In 1921, Drs. Charles H. Mayo (left) and William J. Mayo were made brigadier generals in the army medical reserves. They had enlisted in the reserves between 1912 and 1913. The brothers were prominent in the medical military preparedness movement and alternated duty in Washington, D.C., during World War I.

Base Hospital No. 26

As part of President Woodrow Wilson's "preparedness for peace" program, the Committee of American Physicians for Medical Preparedness was organized in 1916. Dr. William J. Mayo was named chairman and Dr. Charles H. Mayo one of its members. The Committee was later renamed the General Medical Board of the United States Council for National Defense. The Mayos then served as alternate members of its executive committee.

In the fall of 1916, the medical board decided to organize 50 base hospital units. Mayo Clinic was asked to sponsor one of them. Dr. Will felt that because of Mayo's University of Minnesota connection, the university would be the proper sponsoring agent. The Mayo brothers contributed $15,000 toward the new unit's expenses, and enlisted about one-third of its personnel from Rochester. Minneapolis citizens raised a similar amount of money and later donated an equal sum in supplies.

Named Base Hospital No. 26, the unit was ready for mobilization by mid-1917. It was not formally organized until December 10-15, 1917. After training at Fort McPherson, Georgia, the personnel left for France in June 1918. Arriving at Allerey, France, the Minnesota unit was the first on the scene of a center designed to accommodate 10 base hospitals. Members of the Minnesota contingent helped finish the plumbing, wiring, and sewers for the complex.

Surgical work on battle casualties began at the hospital on July 23, 1918. When the other hospital units arrived, Base Hospital No. 26 became solely a surgical facility as the new arrivals took over the GI medical care. Popularly called "the Mayo unit," Base Hospital No. 26 treated 7,200 soldiers before being called home in May 1919. Among its officers were the following from Mayo: Drs. David M. Berkman, James M. Hayes, Oliver C. Melson, Robert D. Mussey, Fred W. Rankin, Thaddeus L. Szlapka, Carl Fisher, Gilbert J. Thomas, and Edward C. Moore.

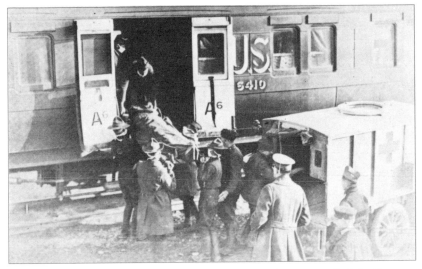

Personnel of Base Hospital 26 unloading the wounded in France during World War I. The Mayo brothers helped organize Base Hospital 26 by contributing funds and enlisting personnel from Rochester. The hospital served at Allerey, France, between 1918 and 1919.

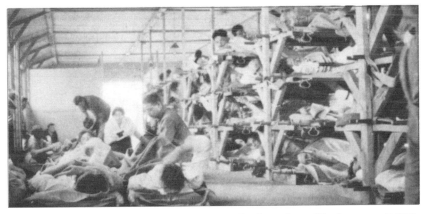

The receiving area for Base Hospital 26 handled some 7,200 soldiers before the unit left France in 1919. Popularly called the Mayo unit, the hospital served as the surgical unit for a center containing 10 hospitals. (*History of Base Hospital 26.*)

Dr. Will's European and Latin American Goodwill Efforts

During his presidency of the American College of Surgeons, 1918 to 1920, Dr. William J. Mayo helped revitalize contacts between European and American physicians. World War I disrupted, and often broke, many of the associations American physicians had enjoyed throughout Europe before the conflict. Dr. Will worked to renew those connections as best he could, considering the state of the economy in Europe.

Dr. Will looked to Latin America as another region in which to improve relations with physicians of his own country. As part of this effort, Dr. Will joined Dr. Franklin H. Martin, secretary of the American College of Surgeons, on a special visit to South America. Their party, including their wives, left New York City by ship in January 1920. Their journey included visits in Argentina, Chile, Jamaica, Peru, Republic of Panama, and Uruguay.

The trip was an instant success. Drs. Mayo and Martin were received in a stately fashion. Welcoming committees greeted them and receptions followed, hosted by government officials and prominent physicians. The visitors toured hospitals, attended clinics, and gave lectures. In several instances, they received honorary degrees and memberships.

After the month-long visit, Dr. Will returned home with a most favorable impression of what he had seen. In his writings about the journey, he found nothing of significance to criticize. He did note, however, the shortage of trained nurses, which resulted from class structures then in effect in the region. There was no middle class from which individuals could be recruited for nursing. Many nurses had been brought in from the United States and Europe.

As a result of Dr. Will's visit, other trips were arranged over the following years for U.S. physicians. The Pan-American Medical Association was organized in 1926, and the Mayo brothers were prominent in its activities. In 1920, Dr. Will wrote, "Whatever may be the after-war responsibility of the United States abroad, we cannot question that our first duty is to develop a sound Pan-Americanism."

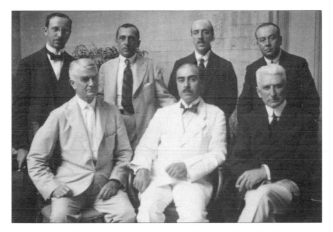

Drs. William J. Mayo and Franklin H. Martin (right) with some physicians in Lima, Peru, on a tour of Latin American medical facilities in 1920. Dr. Will's efforts led to the organization of the Pan-American Medical Association in 1926.

Politics and the Mayo Brothers

As the fame of the Mayo brothers spread, ideas surfaced from time to time promoting their political candidacies. While Dr. Will was away on a South American trip in 1920, a state politician began suggesting that he run for governor on the Democratic ticket. By the time Dr. Will returned home, support for his candidacy was high among Democratic forces.

In a statement to the press, Dr. Will responded:

My opportunity for greatest service lies in another direction . . . My life's work has been wrapped up in the building of the Mayo Clinic, the foundation, and associated endeavors . . . It is a life contract I have set out to fulfill, and I believe the people of this state will bear with me in the belief that I can perform the greatest service to them by holding steady to my purpose.

His response effectively ended political consideration. While the Democrats were disappointed, the Republicans were relieved, admitting that Dr. Will would have been a formidable candidate.

Minnesota politicians did not give up on the Mayo brothers. Four years later, a movement began to nominate Dr. Charlie for President of the United States. It never became widespread, but the idea hung around for some weeks. Dr. Charlie received letters of encouragement from patients, doctors, and even governors of other states supporting his candidacy.

Like his brother, Dr. Charlie refused the draft, although the *New York Times* noted, "He is not so vehement as one would like him to be." Nevertheless, the Mayo brothers did not allow themselves to be drawn into partisan politics. They did, however, have the highest regard for the democratic process.

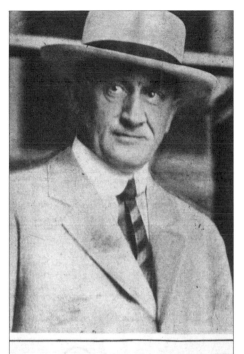

MENTIONED.

Dr. Chas H. Mayo of Rochester who is being pushed forward for the Democratic nomination for president by friends. But he won't run.

In 1924, Dr. Charles H. Mayo was suggested as a presidential candidate. Dr. William J. Mayo had bccn proposed to run for governor in 1920. The brothers did not endorse such efforts, however.(*St. Paul News*, March 23, 1924.)

> All questions in this country can be and should be settled by the ballot box, and in the long run, rightly. As long as public questions are decided without passion or violence by the ballot box our country and our institutions are safe.
>
> *W. J. Mayo*

While the Mayo brothers avoided being political candidates, they were staunch supporters of the democratic process.

Rochester Airport

In July 1928, Harry J. Harwick, Mayo Clinic administrator, announced plans for Mayo to develop a modern airport for Rochester. The 1927 transatlantic flight of Minnesota's Charles A. Lindbergh had created a renewed interest in air transportation. The Mayo brothers recognized the advantages and conveniences that air travel would bring to the Clinic's growing patient population, and they became staunch supporters of airport development in Rochester.

Early in 1928, Rochester Airways opened the first organized airfield in west Rochester. Marshy soil conditions and high operating costs made the new development unfeasible. The Mayo Properties Association (now Mayo Foundation) became interested, and Harwick asked Albert J. Lobb of Mayo's administrative staff to review the local situation. Lobb consulted area engineers and examined several potential sites, including the present airport site, which was then too remote and undeveloped.

These efforts led to incorporation of the Rochester Airport Company as a Mayo Properties Association subsidiary. The new enterprise initially purchased some 284 acres of land on the site of an old racetrack east of the Graham fairgrounds in southeast Rochester. A hangar, shop, and passenger station were constructed, and a passenger service was inaugurated. The fledgling service was taken over by Northwest Airlines in early 1929.

Over the next decade, the Rochester Airport showed a progressive increase in passenger traffic, along with other activities that included a flying school. In 1939, during his last illness, Dr. William J. Mayo expressed concern about the airport needs. As a result, plans for expansion began immediately. An enlarged airport was dedicated on August 4, 1940. It covered 370 acres and featured four paved 3,400-foot runways whose surfaces were comparable to 21 miles of highway; a two-million-candle power beacon on top of the Plummer Building, which could be seen within a 75-mile radius; and radio transmitters in the new passenger terminal for Northwest Airlines' four daily flights. These improvements, along with others, made the Rochester Airport among the finest privately owned airfields of its day.

In 1952, the Rochester Common Council formally named the airport "Lobb Field" in recognition of Albert Lobb's contributions to its development. For nearly a decade more, Lobb Field continued to operate in southeast Rochester until the present Rochester Municipal Airport opened south of the city in 1961.

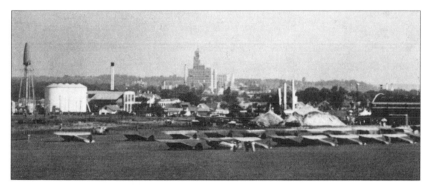

The Rochester airport, looking toward the Clinic. In 1928, Mayo announced plans for the development of a city airport. That same year, the new facility opened in southeast Rochester. Before his death in 1939, Dr. Will requested improvement of the field.

President Roosevelt Visits Rochester

Present-day Mayo people are generally aware of President Franklin D. Roosevelt's visit to Rochester on August 8, 1934, to honor the Mayo brothers.

The occasion is noted on a number of markers in the community. At the northern edge of Soldiers Field golf green, a historic plaque commemorates the location where some 8,000 people gathered under a hot August sun to hear President Roosevelt pay tribute to the Mayo brothers on behalf of the American Legion. The bronze plaque that the President presented is installed in the entryway of the 1928 Plummer Building. In the third-floor historical area of the same building, photographs of the occasion are on prominent display.

Roosevelt's second visit to Rochester, in September 1938, has received less attention, primarily because the President came unofficially as a father awaiting the outcome of surgery on his eldest son, James, at Saint Marys Hospital. The surgery was successful and after a few days, the presidential train left Rochester for Washington. For the brief period, however, Rochester had the distinction of being the "Western White House." At his departure on September 14, 1938, President Roosevelt paid tribute to the Clinic and the people of the community. He said:

Not only am I going away with a full realization of the splendid care that has been taken of my oldest boy (James), the very wonderful work that is being done for humanity as a whole in Rochester, but also I want to thank you for what I can best describe as an understanding heart on the part of the people of Rochester.

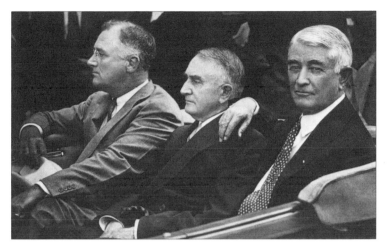

President Roosevelt (left) with the Mayo brothers, Drs. Charles H. Mayo (center) and William J. Mayo. The President came to Rochester in 1934 to honor the brothers on behalf of the American Legion.

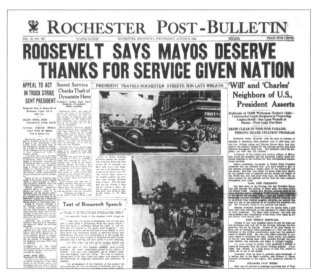

Rochester Post-Bulletin, August 8, 1934.

Mayo Civic Center

With the opening of the enlarged Mayo Civic Center in 1986, a new era of service began for the former Mayo Civic Auditorium. Dr. Charles H. Mayo proposed in early 1938 to build and equip a municipal auditorium for Rochester. The cost of the new structure was to be around $350,000, with Dr. Charlie and Mayo Foundation sharing its expense. Besides providing the community with a meeting place, the building's construction offered Rochester's unemployed the opportunity for much- needed work.

Construction of the Mayo auditorium began later in 1938. Its cornerstone was laid July 28, 1938, with both Mayo brothers participating. In his remarks, Dr. Charlie noted that the project was really a family affair. It was a continuation of the Mayos' interest in city development that dated back several decades before.

When Mayo Civic Auditorium opened in 1939, a series of programs took place on March 8, 9, 10, and 11. The events included a dedication ceremony, an ice revue, a music festival, and a Mardi Gras and follies to introduce the new facility to the community.

The dedication ceremonies held on March 8, 1939, featured local dignitaries, a chorus, and orchestra, along with two rather unusual long-distance communications hookups. The local radio station, KROC, broadcast the proceedings throughout the state via the Northwest Network and also transmitted it to radio station KGAR, in Tucson, Arizona, where the Mayo brothers' winter homes were located.

As part of the dedication ceremonies, Gov. Stassen spoke to the auditorium crowd live from St. Paul via the radio hookup. Dr. Will, representing the Mayo family, also spoke live to the assembly from Tucson using a similar link. At the same time, he and the Mayo family followed the dedicatory exercises in Tucson over what might be called the first teleconference hookup used at Mayo.

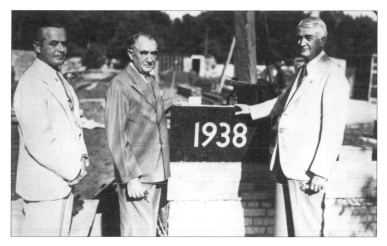

Dr. Charles H. Mayo (center) and Dr. William J. Mayo (right) lay the cornerstone of Mayo Civic Auditorium on July 28, 1938, while Dr. Charlie's son, Dr. Charles W. Mayo, looks on. Dr. Charlie and Mayo Foundation shared in the new building's expense. In 1939, the brothers participated in the opening via a long-distance hookup between Rochester and Tucson, Arizona.

Statues of the Drs. Mayo

With completion of the expanded Mayo Civic Center, the two statues memorializing the Drs. Mayo were given a prominent new location near the entrances.

It was on September 27, 1952, that the Mayo Memorial was originally dedicated in Mayo Park. It featured a tree-lined mall with a statue of the Mayo brothers at one end facing a statue of their father, Dr. W. W. Mayo, at the other.

The eight-foot bronze of the Mayo brothers was executed by internationally known sculptor James Earle Fraser, a Winona native. Born in 1876, he had a distinguished career with a number of his works prominently placed in our nation's capital. He also designed America's widely known Buffalo nickel.

Fraser depicted the Mayo brothers in the surgical gowns they wore in the operating room. The United States commemorative stamp issued in 1964 bore a likeness of the statue.

The statue of Dr. William Worrall Mayo was installed in Mayo Park in 1915. It was sculpted by Leonard Crunelle of Chicago. It was first moved to fit into the memorial plans of 1952.

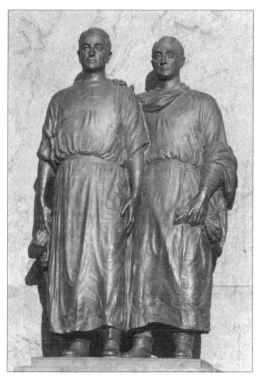

The Mayo brothers' statue in Mayo Park was dedicated in 1952. Executed by James Earle Fraser, the bronze sculpture was relocated to the front entryway of the enlarged Mayo Civic Center in 1986.

Mayo General Hospital

It was the fall of 1943, and in the fields adjoining Galesburg, Illinois, construction was well underway on a new U.S. Army hospital designed to care for the American wounded from World War II. On August 24, 1943, the new facility was named Mayo General Hospital in honor of the Mayo brothers, who had served in World War I.

Mayo General Hospital received its first wounded in February 1944. By the war's end in 1945, more than 14,500 patients had been admitted. The War Department designated the institution as a center for neurosurgery and peripheral vascular diseases. It was equipped with the most modern medical aids of that day.

The hospital complex covered 155 acres. It included 117 redbrick buildings with a bed capacity of 2,350. Complete facilities were provided to make it a self-contained city.

After the war, Mayo General Hospital was closed. Its spacious buildings were used for a time by a branch of the University of Illinois. One of the most recent uses of the physical plant was by the Galesburg Mental Health Center.

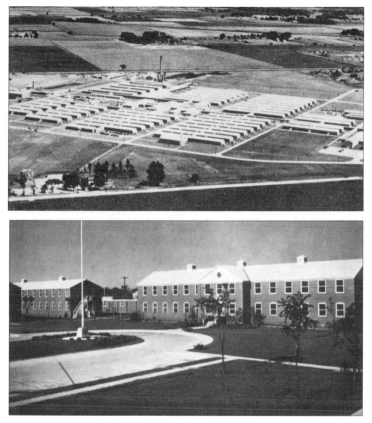

During World War II, the U.S. Army opened Mayo
General Hospital in February 1944. It was named after
the Mayo brothers and covered 155 acres of land near
Galesburg, Illinois. The facility featured 117 buildings
with a 2,300-bed capacity.

S.S. *Mayo Brothers*

During World War II, the name "Liberty" was assigned to a class of emergency cargo ships that played an important role in supplying American troops overseas. During the conflict, more than 2,700 such vessels were built. Initially, it required 243 days to complete a ship. As the end of the war neared, one could be launched in a week.

Early in the war, the Delta Shipbuilding Company constructed a Liberty ship named the S.S. *Mayo Brothers*. It was their 28th vessel of this type. The launching took place on December 14, 1942, in New Orleans.

Three Minnesota high-school students officiated at the ceremonies. As winners of the state's scrap-metal drive, they represented Minnesota at the christening. Cecile Carlson of Wolverton, Minnesota, broke the traditional champagne bottle over the ship's bow before it slid sideways into the water. Her student companions were Edgar Pierce of Staples and Roy Brandt of Olivia, Minnesota.

The ship's name was the suggestion of Minnesota students. Besides Mayo, Alexander Ramsey (first governor of the Minnesota Territory) and Henry H. Sibley (first governor of the state) had been nominated. The maritime commission made the final name selection.

Like other Liberty ships, the S.S. *Mayo Brothers* was 441 feet, six inches long. It had a deadweight carrying capacity of more than 10,000 tons. After the war, the ship was put into the National Defense Reserve Fleet at Mobile, Alabama. A few of these vessels saw active duty during the Korean conflict. A few years later, the reserve ships, including the Mayo ship, were sold for scrap. Thus ended a career of service for the vessel that had carried men and materials in at least two major theaters of operations in the South Pacific and Omaha Beach during World War II.

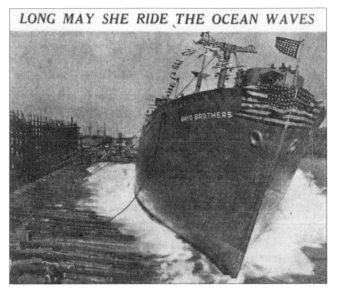

LONG MAY SHE RIDE THE OCEAN WAVES

In December 1942, the S.S. *Mayo Brothers* was launched in New Orleans. The Liberty ship served in the South Pacific and Omaha Beach during World War II. It was christened by three Minnesota high-school students.

Mayo Memorial at the University of Minnesota

On October 21-22, 1954, dedication ceremonies took place for the Mayo Memorial on the main campus of the University of Minnesota in Minneapolis. Named in honor of the Mayo brothers, the impressive building features a 16-story tower with three six-story wings that connect the university hospital and medical school buildings.

Shortly after the Mayo brothers died in 1939, Gov. Harold E. Stassen appointed a Mayo Memorial Commission, composed of outstanding Minnesotans, to decide upon a suitable memorial. Dr. Will had served as a member of the Board of Regents of the University for 32 years. Dr. Charlie had also served for many years as Professor of Surgery. They had been a vital force in the development of medicine on the university campus.

In 1943, the Minnesota legislature resolved to participate in the memorial to the brothers who brought Minnesota "enduring fame." The Committee of Founders was appointed by Gov. Edward J. Thye. Donald J. Cowling, retired president of Carleton College, headed the group. The committee proposed construction of a building to help centralize the medical school facilities of the University of Minnesota. After a series of delays, construction began in the summer of 1950. Unfortunately, steel shortages caused by the Korean War intervened, and the building was not completely enclosed until 1953.

With the dedication of the Mayo Memorial in 1954, the university had what some called a "campus in the clouds." The building was the tallest on campus and opened when university attendance exceeded 20,000 students for the first time.

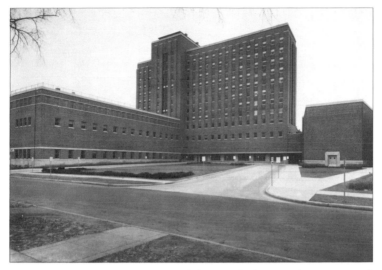

The Mayo Memorial Building of the University of Minnesota Medical Center opened in 1954. The tallest building on the university campus, it was nicknamed a "campus in the clouds."

Stamp Honoring the Drs. Mayo

A temporary U.S. Postal substation was set up on September 11, 1964, in the main lobby of the Mayo Building to sell the first "Doctors Mayo" commemorative postage stamps and provide "First Day of Issue" cancellations for the stamp. The location was one of several in Rochester that made the stamp available on that date. Nationwide sales of the balance of the initial 120 million printing of the medical stamp began the following day.

The issuance of the Mayo stamp culminated the efforts of a citizens' committee and several individuals. Beginning in 1957, Clarence Stearns, a long-time Rochester photographer and friend of the Mayo brothers, began encouraging prominent friends to urge the U.S. Post Office to issue a Mayo brothers' commemorative stamp. Stearns enlisted a small group of interested people before he turned the project over to Roy Watson, Jr., president of the Kahler Corporation. Watson expanded the group to form a committee of noted citizens in favor of the stamp. Their efforts were successful, and in April 1964 the government announced the Mayo brothers' stamp.

As part of the first day of issuance events, U.S. Postmaster General John A. Gronouski came to Rochester to dedicate the new stamp. R. Putnam Kingsbury, Mayo administrator and stamp enthusiast, headed the local committee making dedication arrangements. During the ceremonies, Gronouski said the stamp was "a tribute from a grateful nation for the good works of those men . . . they left us a medical legacy of genius and generosity." He presented Mayo family representatives and others with albums of the new stamp.

The Rochester Stamp Club, headed by Charles W. Tannert, prepared the official cachet envelope for the stamp. The cachet's design was executed by John M. Hutcheson, Mayo medical illustrator. The club also sponsored a well-attended regional stamp show to coincide with the event.

The commemorative stamp depicts the heads of the Mayo brothers, based upon the statue by James Earle Fraser that now stands in front of Mayo Civic Center. Victor S. McCloskey, Jr., modeled the design, which included the staff of Aesculapius, Greco-Roman god of medicine. The stamp was printed in green, the symbolic color of medicine.

During the first day sale in Rochester, the post office handled some 500,000 covers. Today, copies of the stamp affixed to a first day cover have become collectors' items.

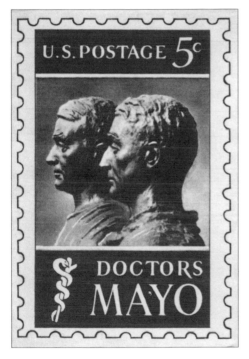

Artistic rendering of commemorative stamp, first issued on September 11, 1964, in Rochester, Minnesota. A citizens' committee and several individuals, whose efforts dated back to 1957, were responsible for the stamp's issuance.

· SECTION III ·

Development of Mayo Clinic and Mayo Foundation

Around the turn of the century, the Mayo brothers began forming in Rochester the integrated private group practice of medicine known as Mayo Clinic. The roots of this innovative multispecialty practice extended back several decades to the family's pioneer medical practice. With the increased numbers of patients and the subsequent addition of clinical, surgical, laboratory, and administrative associates, the basic organizational aspects of Mayo Clinic and Mayo Foundation were formalized between 1914 and 1923.

The Mayo Institutions

The success of the Drs. Mayo and their partners in Rochester laid a firm foundation for continuing work in medical practice, education, and research. Recognizing their obligations to the future, the Mayo brothers set up institutions between 1915 and 1919 by which these activities could grow and develop years after the brothers' personal participation had ceased.

In a series of steps beginning in 1915, the Mayo brothers developed America's first graduate program in clinical medicine. They endowed the activity at first with $1.5 million that had been carefully saved from their accumulated earnings and investments of more than 25 years' duration. The program was initially affiliated with the University of Minnesota. Its educational and research opportunities had been developed much earlier by the Mayos in their internships and laboratory facilities.

Since its formation, the program has steadily grown, and today numbers around 10,000 alumni scattered throughout the world. Its concepts still continue, but in 1964, it became known as Mayo Graduate School of Medicine. In 1983, the school became independent, no longer affiliated with the University of Minnesota.

One other event occurred in the 1915-1919 period that made Mayo Clinic secure for future generations. On October 8, 1919, Drs. William J. and Charles H. Mayo signed the deed of gift that conveyed all of the physical properties and assets of Mayo Clinic to Mayo Properties Association. The event climaxed the work of a committee established in 1918 by the Mayo brothers. Its members, Harry J. Harwick, Judge George Granger, and Burt W. Eaton, carefully worked out the agreement that remains today.

Through the years, the purposes of the deed have remained essentially unchanged. The name Mayo Properties Association was later shortened to Mayo Association, and, in 1964, changed to Mayo Foundation.

Following the incorporation of Mayo Properties Association in

1919, the Mayo brothers developed an organizational structure for the Clinic that would guide it into the future. Initially, the brothers established the Board of Governors, charged with the operation of the Clinic. Shortly thereafter, the Mayos instituted a system of committees responsible for specific areas within the Clinic. The committees reported regularly to the Board on their actions and deliberations.

Membership on the committees came primarily from the medical staff. Through such committee activities, members learned about Clinic operations and later became candidates for appointment to the Board of Governors.

At first, the brothers served the Board as its leaders. In 1932, they stepped down from the Board of Governors, and Dr. Donald C. Balfour became chairman. Since then, Drs. Robert D. Mussey (1937-1946), Arlie R. Barnes (1947-1952), Samuel F. Haines (1953-1956), James T. Priestley II (1957-1963), L. Emmerson Ward (1964-1975), and W. Eugene Mayberry (1976-1987), have served.

Dr. Robert R. Waller is the current chairman of Mayo Clinic Rochester Board of Governors as well as chief executive officer of Mayo Foundation. Mayo Clinic Jacksonville Board of Governors is chaired by Dr. Leo F. Black, and Mayo Clinic Scottsdale Board of Governors is chaired by Dr. Richard W. Hill.

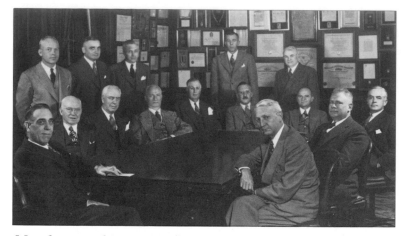

Members and past members of the Board of Governors, Mayo Clinic, photographed in December 1947. Standing left: James T. Priestley II (Board chairman, 1957-1963); Howard K. Gray; Lawrence M. Randall; J. William Harwick; and Albert J. Lobb. Seated left: Arlie R. Barnes (Board chairman 1947-1952); Robert D. Mussey (Board chairman, 1937-1946); Melvin S. Henderson; Donald C. Balfour (Board chairman, 1933-1936); Harry J. Harwick; Samuel F. Haines (Board chairman, 1953-1956); Waltman Walters; Charles W. Mayo; Frank C. Mann; and David M. Berkman.

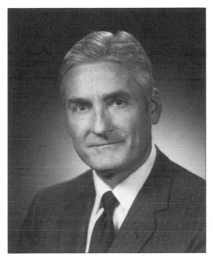

Dr. L. Emmerson Ward
Board chairman, 1964-1975.

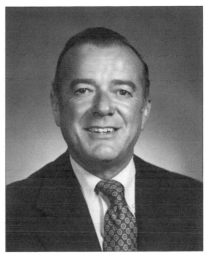

Dr. W. Eugene Mayberry
Board chairman, 1976-1987.

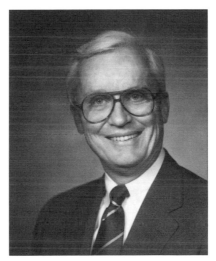

Dr. Robert R. Waller
Current Board chairman.

Origins of "Mayo Clinic"

Who first used the name, "Mayo Clinic"? Surprisingly, it did not originate within the Clinic, but rather came from the medical profession. Initially, the Mayo brothers included each partner's name in their firm's title.

As physicians came to Rochester to see the Mayos operate, they frequently referred to their destination as "the Mayo Brothers' Clinic" or "Mayos' Clinic." The railroads and patients quickly made these shorter references popular. However, the partnership name remained until the 1914 Building was erected, and establishment of Mayo's educational program and foundation made the name "Mayo Clinic" correct.

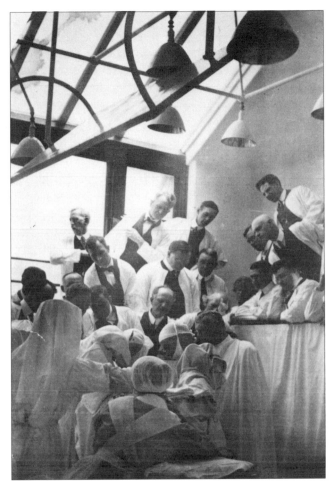

As physicians and surgeons flocked to Rochester to see the Mayo brothers at work in surgery, they frequently spoke of "Mayos' Clinic" or "the Mayo Brothers' Clinic" as their destination. The railroads and patients soon popularized this name, and in 1914 Mayo adopted it.

The Mayo Partnership

The partnership era of the Mayo practice begin in 1892, when Dr. Augustus W. Stinchfield, a well-known practitioner from Eyota, Minnesota, joined the Mayos as their first partner. Two years later, Christopher Graham, brother-in-law of Dr. Charlie Mayo, received his medical degree and joined the growing practice as the second partner.

With the retirement of Dr. Stinchfield in 1906, Drs. Melvin C. Millet and Henry S. Plummer became members of the partnership. Both were natives of the Racine, Minnesota, area. Dr. Millet had been associated with the Mayos since 1899 and Dr. Plummer since 1901.

The untimely death of Dr. Millet in 1907 cut short his promising career in urology. Later that year, he was succeeded in the partnership by Dr. E. Starr Judd. A Rochester native, Dr. Judd had begun practicing with the group in 1902.

In 1915, Dr. Donald C. Balfour became the last member of the Mayo partnership. Dr. Balfour arrived in Rochester from Canada in 1907. With the retirement of Dr. Graham in 1919, and establishment of the Mayo Properties Association (forerunner of Mayo Foundation) by the remaining partners that year, the modern era of the Mayo medical practice began.

The Mayo partnership was only a participating arrangement in which each member shared a percentage of that year's income. The Mayos retained ownership of the property and its assets.

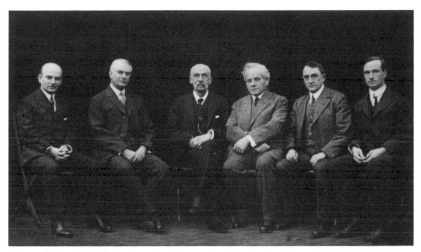

Some of the Mayo partners, photographed with Sir Rickman Godlee, president of the Royal College of Surgeons, in Rochester around 1913. From left: Drs. E. Starr Judd, William J. Mayo, Sir Rickman Godlee, Drs. Christopher Graham, Charles H. Mayo, and Donald C. Balfour, Sr.

Dr. Stinchfield: the First Mayo Partner

Augustus White Stinchfield, the first partner of the Drs. Mayo, was born on December 21, 1842, in Phillips, Maine. After a teaching experience in Wisconsin and service in the Civil War, he received his Doctor of Medicine degree in 1868 from Bowdoin College, Maine.

Dr. Stinchfield returned to the West to practice in Verona, Missouri, from 1869 to 1872, when he moved to Dundas, Minnesota. In the fall of 1873, he relocated his practice in Eyota, Minnesota. During the 19 years that Dr. Stinchfield practiced there, he was preceptor for at least eight young men who became well-qualified physicians.

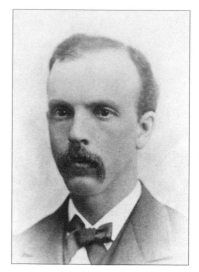

First partner of the Drs. Mayo, Dr. Augustus W. Stinchfield was a noted area physician. He joined the firm in 1892 and retired in 1906.

In February 1892, he accepted an invitation from the Mayos to become their first partner. During his association with them, he focused his attention on the diagnosis and treatment of diseases of the heart and lungs. In 1906, he retired from the firm.

On May 1, 1878, Dr. Stinchfield married Martha Jane Bear. They had five children, one of whom was a boy who died in his youth from a railway accident. Three of their daughters married Mayo physicians: Nellie became the wife of Dr. William F. Braasch; Lura married Dr. Henry W. Meyerding; and Alice married Dr. Mark J. Anderson.

Dr. Stinchfield died in Rochester on March 15, 1917, during his 75th year.

Dr. Graham: the Second Mayo Partner

Christopher Graham, the second partner of the Drs. Mayo, was born on April 3, 1856, near Truxton, Cortland County, New York. He was sixth of the 13 children born to Joseph Graham and Jane Twentyman Graham.

About a month after his birth, the family left New York by horse-drawn wagon for Minnesota. They settled about five miles northwest of Rochester at Grahamholm. The elder Graham farmed there for some 40 years before retiring in Rochester.

The Graham household experienced many hardships of Minnesota pioneer life. The father was a steadfast worker whose

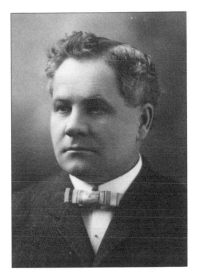

Dr. Christopher Graham, the second Mayo partner, trained initially as a veterinarian. He joined the Mayos in 1894 and retired as head of the Division of Medicine in 1919.

precept helped the family overcome the lack of means or opportunity. Mrs. Graham had a talent for aiding and comforting the sick. She nursed all who needed her, without material gain. Her children later estimated that she had assisted in the birth of 243 babies, without medical advice and without losing a mother or child.

Christopher's sisters, Dinah and Edith, followed their mother's example and became professional nurses. Dinah Frances Graham was the first anesthetist at Saint Marys Hospital. After her marriage, Edith Maria Graham became anesthetist and trained the Sisters of Saint Francis in nursing at the hospital. She later married Dr. Charles H. Mayo.

"Kit," as Christopher Graham was more commonly known, obtained his education through years of persistent effort. After the minimal district school education, he finally secured some private tutoring in Rochester during his 21st year. This four-month experience enabled him to teach district school during the winter months. In 1882, he entered the University of Minnesota as a special student. Five years later, he received his Bachelor of Science degree at the age of 26. From 1887-89, he taught at Shattuck School in Faribault, Minnesota.

Christopher Graham entered the University of Pennsylvania as a veterinary medicine major in 1889 and graduated in 1892. After he served a year as veterinarian with the University of Minnesota Experiment Station, his strong interest in clinical medicine won out and, with the Mayo brothers' encouragement, he returned to the University of Pennsylvania, where he received the Doctor of Medicine degree in 1894 at the age of 38.

Dr. Graham returned to Rochester as the first intern at Saint Marys Hospital. After becoming the Mayos' second partner, Christopher Graham grew in professional stature. He became highly regarded as an internist and diagnostician with special interest in diseases of the digestive tract.

In 1914, Dr. Graham became head of the Division of Medicine of Mayo Clinic. His retirement in 1919 ended 25 years of productive life at Mayo. Dr. Graham's retirement, however, did not end his long-time involvement in farming, horticulture, and animal husbandry. He continued to achieve in these fields, receiving numerous honors. His support of the Olmsted County Fair Association led to generous gifts of real estate to the association and to the City of Rochester.

Christopher Graham married Elizabeth Blanche Brackenridge on January 4, 1899. They enlarged and beautified the pioneer Brackenridge home in southeast Rochester, where they lived throughout their lives. Dr. Graham died June 20, 1952, in Rochester, during his 96th year.

Dr. Millet:
the Third Mayo Partner

Melvin C. Millet, the third partner of the Mayos, was born on September 22, 1868, near Hamilton in Sumner Township, Fillmore County, Minnesota. He was the son of Mr. and Mrs. Roscoe G. Millet, and one of four children. He spent his first 21 years in Sumner, attending district school and working the family farm.

Interested in a profession, Melvin graduated from Winona Teachers College and taught district school for a year. Encouraged by his uncle, he became Dr. Rollo C. Dugan's assistant in Dover, Minnesota. In 1892, he entered the University of Minnesota, where he received the M.D. degree, with high honors, in June 1895.

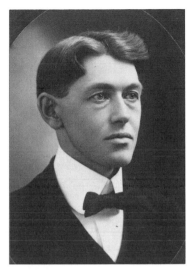

Dr. Melvin C. Millet joined the Mayos in 1898. He laid the foundation for Mayo's Section on Urology before his untimely death in 1907.

Initially, Dr. Millet practiced in Dover in place of Dr. Dugan, who had moved to Eyota to take Dr. Stinchfield's place after he left for the Mayo practice. Finding the Dover people "too rascally healthy," Dr. Millet joined his old friend Dr. Milan J. Hart in Le Roy, Minnesota. In November 1898, Dr. Millet became a resident physician with the Mayos at Saint Marys Hospital.

With the Mayos, Dr. Millet expanded his interest in gastric analysis to include renal disease. He became one of the first to use and advocate the direct-view cystoscope. His work in urology laid the foundation for Mayo's Section on Urology. Besides Dr. Millet's involvement in these activities, he displayed a special interest in diseases of children. Dr. Henry S. Plummer, his second cousin, credited Dr. Millet with recognizing the changes that were coming in the treatment of childhood diseases.

When Dr. Augustus W. Stinchfield retired from the Mayo partnership on July 1, 1906, Drs. Melvin C. Millet and Henry S. Plummer became partners in the firm. Dr. Plummer had already joined Mayo in 1901.

Unfortunately, Dr. Millet's promising career was cut short by his death from Bright's disease on May 7, 1907. He was 39 years old. Dr. Millet's wife, the former Mary A. Frick, later married John L. Magaw of Rochester.

Dr. Millet's only child, Roscoe Frick Millet, became a physician. He served a fellowship at Mayo from 1930 to 1934 and died in 1979.

Dr. Plummer: the Fourth Mayo Partner

On March 3, 1874, Henry Stanley Plummer was born in Hamilton, Minnesota. He was one of four children of Dr. Albert and Isabelle Steer Plummer. Both his sister, Sadie, and his brother, Ray, died in infancy. Henry and his remaining younger brother, William Albert, later became physicians associated with Mayo Clinic.

Dr. Albert Plummer, Henry's father, grew up in New Hampshire. After serving in the Civil War, the elder Plummer attended medical school at Bowdoin College in Maine, graduating in 1867. Deciding to move west, Dr. Albert Plummer arrived penniless and on foot in Hamilton, Minnesota, in 1869, to begin a successful medical career lasting 24 years in that community.

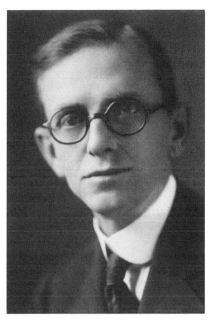

Dr. Henry S. Plummer, the fourth Mayo partner, was the son of a prominent physician. He joined the firm in 1901. Before his death in 1936, he left Mayo with a rich legacy in medicine, engineering, and architecture.

In his youth, Henry Plummer assisted his father's medical practice, much as the Mayo brothers helped their father. In 1898, Henry S. Plummer received the M.D. degree from Northwestern University in Chicago. He returned home to join his father in practice in Racine, Minnesota. His father had relocated there in 1893.

Dr. Plummer spent only three years with his father, because a professional visit by Dr. Will Mayo to Racine brought young Dr.

Plummer's capabilities to the Mayos' attention. Impressed by Dr. Plummer's knowledge of blood, the Mayo brothers invited him to Rochester in 1901 to develop their clinical laboratories.

Dr. H. S. Plummer's arrival launched a career that was varied and full of accomplishment in the growing firm of Drs. Mayo, Stinchfield, and Graham. He made contributions to hematology, roentgenology, bronchoscopy, esophagoscopy, electrocardiography, and to knowledge of the physiology and pathology of the thyroid gland.

His system for Mayo's medical records remains in use today. Dr. Plummer contributed significantly to the development of the Clinic's communication system. His understanding of the needs of Mayo's medical practice and his knowledge of architecture and engineering culminated in the design and construction of the 1914 Mayo Clinic Building and the 1928 Clinic building that bears his name. Dr. Plummer became a partner in 1906. He was an incorporator and a member of the board of Mayo Properties Association (today's Mayo Foundation). He also was an original member of the Mayo Clinic Board of Governors.

Dr. Plummer's marriage to Daisy M. Berkman in 1904 strengthened his interest in art, literature, music, and horticulture. Their attractive home in southwest Rochester remains a tribute to their cultural pursuits.

On December 31, 1936, Dr. Henry S. Plummer died from cerebral thrombosis. When he became ill earlier that afternoon, he recognized the symptoms of his affliction and correctly predicted the rapid course his condition would take.

Dr. Judd:
the Fifth Mayo Partner

Edward Starr Judd was the fifth partner in the Mayo practice. Starr, as he was known, was born in Rochester, Minnesota, on July 11, 1878, the son of Edward Francis Judd and Emma Jane Myers. His parents were born in Connecticut of pioneer families.

Looking for a more healthful climate, Starr's father came to Rochester in 1869 and became a successful grain buyer. The elder Judd's marriage in Rochester produced four children. The two girls died in infancy, as did their father not long after. Starr and his brother, Cornelius, were reared by their mother.

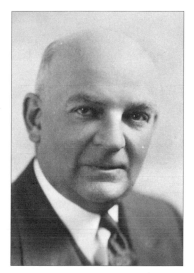

Dr. E. Starr Judd was a Rochester native. He joined the Mayos in 1902 and became a leading surgeon before his death from pneumonia in 1935.

E. Starr Judd was educated in the local public schools, where he became captain of the Rochester High School football team in 1897. During his high school days, he worked odd jobs at Saint Marys Hospital. This exposure helped him select medicine for his career at the University of Minnesota.

In 1902, E. Starr Judd received his M.D. degree and returned to Rochester to begin an internship at Saint Marys Hospital. In 1903, he became first assistant to Dr. Charlie in surgery. His talent for surgery and industrious manner soon led to his appointment as head of his own surgical section at Mayo in 1904. At the age of 26, he became the first person to help the Mayo brothers handle their heavy surgical load. For the next 31 years, Dr. Judd's skill as a master in general surgery brought him numerous achievements.

With the death of Dr. Melvin Millet in 1907, Dr. Judd became a partner in the Mayo firm. Later he became an original member of the Clinic's Board of Governors. He also was an incorporator and a member of the board of Mayo Properties Association.

Among his honors, Dr. Judd was president of the American Medical Association (1931), the Minnesota State Medical Association (1923), the Western Surgical Association (1929), and the Society of Clinical Surgery (1932). During World War I, he served as major and director of the School of Instruction for officers and enlisted men at Rochester. Later he became lieutenant colonel in the U.S. Army Reserves.

E. Starr Judd married Helen Berkman on September 12, 1908. They had five children. Among them were Dr. Edward S. Judd, a Mayo surgeon who retired in 1976; and Dr. David B. Judd, a Mayo surgical fellow in 1946 and, before his death, a surgeon in Eugene, Oregon.

While on a trip, E. Starr Judd became ill with a virulent pneumonia and died November 30, 1935, in Chicago. Mayo alumni established the Judd-Plummer Lectureship at Mayo to honor Dr. Judd and his brother-in-law, Dr. Henry S. Plummer. In 1958, land near Country Club Manor was given to Rochester for Starr Judd Park.

Dr. Balfour: the Sixth Mayo Partner

The last partner to join the Mayo practice was Donald Church Balfour, M.D. His distinguished career at Mayo spanned 40 years of accomplishment in surgery and education.

Dr. Balfour was born in Toronto, Ontario, Canada, on August 22, 1882, the son of Walter Balfour and Alice Church Balfour. Growing up in Hamilton, Ontario, young Balfour obtained his preliminary education at the Hamilton Collegiate Institute. He received his Bachelor of Medicine from the University of Toronto in 1906.

During his internship at Hamilton General Hospital, Dr. Balfour was influenced by Dr. Ingersoll Olmsted, a prominent

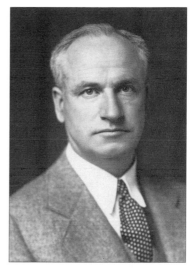

Dr. Donald C. Balfour, Sr., the last partner of the Drs. Mayo, was a Canadian. He joined the Mayos in 1907 and became noted as a surgeon and an educator before his retirement in 1947.

surgeon and teacher, to choose surgery as his specialty. After a medical school friend, Dr. M. S. Henderson, mentioned an opening in pathology at Mayo, Dr. Balfour promptly left Canada for Rochester. When he arrived at Mayo on July 7, 1907, his appointment as an assistant in pathology was waiting for him. A telegram from Dr. Olmsted had already apprised the Mayos of Balfour's potential.

After a year in surgical pathology, working with Drs. Louis B. Wilson and W. C. MacCarty, Dr. Balfour became a clinical assistant in 1908, working with Dr. Christopher Graham.

In 1909, Dr. Balfour became a junior surgeon rotating between the surgical services of the Mayo brothers and Drs. E. Starr Judd and Emil H. Beckman. In 1912, Dr. Balfour became head of a section of surgery. For the next 35 years, he became internationally known for his skills in surgery. He devised various instruments and equipment for the operating room. As a general surgeon, he was involved in a variety of surgical procedures, with special interest in diseases of the stomach and duodenum.

Dr. Balfour was a strong supporter of Mayo's programs in education and research. In 1935, he became associate director of what is today's Mayo Graduate School of Medicine and its director from 1937 until his retirement in 1947.

In 1915, Dr. Balfour became the last person to join the Mayo partnership. Later, he played a prominent role in the evolution of the Mayo institutions that replaced the partnership. He was an original member of the Board of Governors of Mayo Clinic and chairman from 1933 to 1936. He was also an incorporator and member of Mayo Properties Association board (today's Mayo Foundation).

Among his many honors and memberships was the presidency of the American College of Surgeons in 1935. He was a recipient of the Friedenwald Medal, American Gastroenterological Association; Distinguished Service Award, American Medical Association; cross of Knight Commander of the Royal Order of the Crown of Italy; and insigne of commander in the Order of Merit of the Republic of Chile. Among his honorary fellowships were those from the Royal Colleges of Surgeons in England, Scotland, Australasia, and Canada. He received honorary degrees from six colleges and universities. In his honor, Balfour Hall in Mayo Foundation House was dedicated in 1947, and the Donald Church Balfour Visiting Professorship was established in 1960 at Mayo.

Dr. Balfour married Carrie L. Mayo (Dr. Will's eldest daughter) on May 28, 1910. The Balfours were active supporters of the arts, with a special interest in music. They had four children. Among them were Mary Damon (deceased), who married Dr. H. Frederic Helmholz, Jr., Mayo Emeritus Staff; and Drs. William M. Balfour (Lawrence, Kansas) and Donald C. Balfour, Jr. (deceased), who completed Mayo residencies. Dr. Donald C. Balfour passed away in Rochester, Minnesota, on July 25, 1963, of pulmonary edema caused by myocardial infarction.

The First Clinic Business Manager

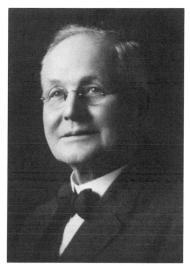

William Beck Graham was the first business manager of Mayo Clinic. He was the eldest son of 13 children born to Joseph Graham and Jane Twentyman Graham.

Their parents came to America from England with their respective families in the 1840s. After their marriage in 1847, the Grahams settled in Cortland County, New York, where William was born on July 13, 1848. Eight years later, the family headed west, arriving in Rochester by covered wagon in 1856.

William Beck Graham was the first business manager of the Mayo firm. An area businessman, he joined the Mayos in 1901.

The Grahams settled on a farm known as Grahamholm in Kalmar Township, Olmsted County, five miles northwest of the city. After William attended Spring's school in Rochester, he was a cheese and butter maker. He became an overseer of cheese factories and creameries in Rochester and St. Paul for some 15 years. He married Grace Morrow in 1873, and they celebrated their 60th wedding anniversary in 1933.

Graham became business manager for the Drs. Mayo in March 1901. The medical practice had recently moved into the Masonic Temple Building in downtown Rochester. During his tenure, Graham helped develop the business office of the Clinic. After the opening of the Mayo Clinic Building in 1914, he continued to press for improved business practices. In his senior years, he regularly visited the office, continuing his visits until two years before his death on January 31, 1940. The Graham Building, 425 Third Avenue, Southwest, was named to honor him and other members of the Graham family.

Mayo Administration and H. J. Harwick

Harry J. Harwick holds a prominent place among those who made many significant contributions to the growth and development of Mayo Clinic.

Associated with Mayo from 1908 until 1952, Harwick was the key figure in developing the concept of lay administration at the institution. As a protege of Dr. William J. Mayo, he fostered the evolution of medical administration as an enhancement to group practice that frees the physician from the daily burdens of routine business affairs.

Because of Harwick's efforts, lay administration became an important component of the integrated group practice of medicine that the Mayo brothers pioneered in Rochester, Minnesota.

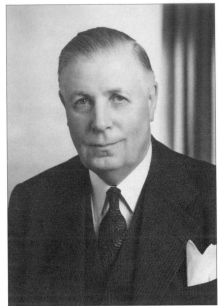

Harry J. Harwick joined the Mayo business office in 1908. He pioneered the concept of lay administration at Mayo and became chairman of the Department of Administration before his retirement in 1952.

Harwick joined the growing Mayo practice on his 21st birthday, September 2, 1908. With his parents, he came to Rochester from Winona, Minnesota, two years before and had found employment with the First National Bank as a teller. He later recalled that he learned the banking business from the ground up by doing a variety of jobs, including shoveling snow and sweeping the floors. He was happy in the world of banking and accounting and hoped to make a successful career in it.

Despite overtures that offered him challenges in banks

elsewhere, Harwick elected to stay in Rochester and grow with the community. His opportunity came in 1908, when the Mayo brothers needed an assistant to William Graham in their business office. Dr. Will hired Harwick for the post.

Graham had headed the Mayos' business operations since 1901. He was a mature man with considerable business experience and service as city justice. When Harwick was appointed, Graham was managing the Mayos' business affairs in a room in their diagnostic offices in downtown Rochester. The offices were then located in the original Masonic Temple Building, which the Mayos had financially helped to erect.

After he was hired, Harwick assisted Graham in routine business office matters. He also began to modernize the accounting system, as Dr. Will had suggested when he was employed. In consultation with Graham, Harwick introduced a ledger card system to replace the ledger system then in vogue. The new approach had merit, but its acceptance by all concerned was less than wholehearted. Harwick found a valuable ally in Dr. Henry S. Plummer, one of the newer appointees to the Mayo medical staff.

In 1907, Dr. Plummer had introduced his new unit medical record system to the Mayo practice. He was also meeting some opposition in this undertaking and was happy to join forces with Harwick in promoting their innovations. Their joint efforts were successful, and the new programs were instituted.

The new accounting scheme was only the beginning for Harwick at Mayo. During his more than four decades at Mayo Clinic, he helped to establish Mayo Foundation and develop the financial stability of Mayo and its enterprises. After the death of the Mayo brothers in 1939, he was appointed the Chief Executive Officer of the Mayo Board. Harwick retired from Mayo in 1952 and died on February 11, 1978. The Harwick Building at Mayo was named in his honor when it opened in 1961.

Following Harwick's retirement, Mayo administration has been headed by G. Slade Schuster (1952-70), J. William Harwick (1970-76), Robert C. Roesler (1976-82) and, currently, Robert W. Fleming.

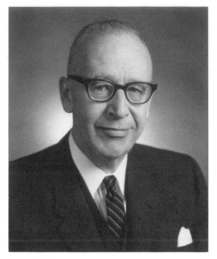

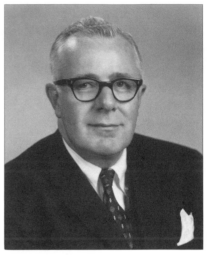

G. Slade Schuster
Administration
Chairman, 1952-1970.

J. William Harwick
Administration
Chairman, 1970-1976.

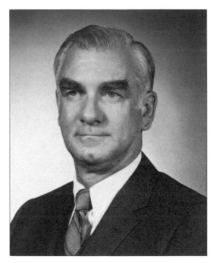

Robert C. Roesler
Administration
Chairman, 1976-1982.

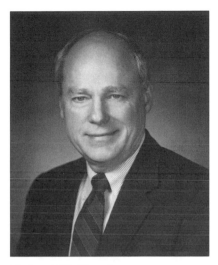

Robert W. Fleming
Administration
Chairman, 1982 to present.

Mayo's Legal Department

The Legal Department at Mayo had its origins in the activities of Burt W. Eaton, pioneer Rochester attorney. Around 1900, Eaton became the Mayo brothers' financial advisor and the attorney who handled their legal matters, including the early partnership agreements. During his early days of law practice, Eaton's partner was Frank B. Kellogg, who later went to Washington as U.S. Secretary of State.

In 1917, the Mayo brothers persuaded Judge George W. Granger to resign his district judgeship and become their legal counsel for several years while he helped Harry J. Harwick work out the details of the Clinic's reorganization plan. Granger had previously assisted with the legalities of establishing Mayo Graduate School of Medicine in 1915. Judge Granger's counsel helped in the 1919 formation of Mayo Properties Association, today's Mayo Foundation.

On September 1, 1925, Albert J. Lobb became Mayo's legal counsel and a member of the administrative section. Before coming to the Clinic, Lobb had been active at the University of Minnesota as a faculty member, presidential assistant, comptroller, and secretary to the Board of Regents. While in Rochester, he became an expert on medicolegal problems and lectured regularly on the topic. Lobb served as secretary-treasurer of Mayo Foundation, 1939-51, and as the first president of the Rochester Airport Company. Lobb Field in southeast Rochester was named after him in 1952.

After Lobb's retirement in 1949, Harry A. Blackmun joined Mayo's administrative section in 1950 as legal counsel. He became a founder of the Rochester Methodist Hospital and the author of its original articles of incorporation. Blackmun remained with Mayo until his appointment as a federal judge in 1959. Later, he continued his rise to national prominence with an associate justice appointment to the U.S. Supreme Court in 1970.

Between 1960-62, Gregg Orwoll served as Mayo's associate legal counsel after succeeding A. M. (Sandy) Keith. Orwoll was named legal counsel and chairman of the department in 1963. The current chairman, Robert M. Moore, Jr., assumed his responsibilities in 1987.

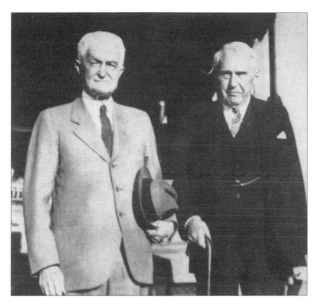

Burt W. Eaton (left) and his early law partner,
Frank B. Kellogg, later U.S. Secretary of State.
Eaton was Mayo's first legal and financial
advisor, beginning around 1900.

Beginnings of General Service

One of the earliest sectional groups in the Clinic is General Service. Its origins can be traced back to Jay Neville and John "Jack" Craig, the "hired men" of the pioneer Mayo family.

The custom of "hiring out" was common on the American frontier, and many people began their employment through such an arrangement. Usually, such people lived with the employing family and often became closely associated with their daily activities. Neville and Craig began their careers with Dr. William Worrall Mayo in their early twenties. They remained with members of the Mayo family for the rest of their lives.

Jay Neville, a Civil War veteran, was initially in charge of the Mayo farm in southeast Rochester. He took a personal interest in the growing Mayo children, including Will and Charlie. After Dr. Will and Hattie were married and moved to College Street (Fourth Street, Southwest), Neville joined them and remained with them for 24 years.

With the opening of Mayo offices in the first Masonic Temple Building, Jay Neville became the general handyman there. Among his many duties was the filing of Clinic correspondence. At first, he merely pasted the letters end to end and rolled them up like a scroll to fit a cylinder. In time, Neville learned of drugstore prescription practices and applied his version of them by using a piece of wire or heavy twine on which to group the letters as he received them.

Jay Neville was a devoted member of the Mayo family and their medical practice. His colorful personality made him a familiar and lovable figure to Mayo patients and staff alike.

Neville's contemporary, "Jack" Craig, was responsible for handling the Mayo horses. In days prior to the automobile, he was a frequent sight with his beautiful bays outside the Mayo offices or the hospitals. He often helped Clinic staff get to distant homes on wintry days or carried small parties off on sleigh rides in the crisp winter air.

The pride and care that these early "general service" people demonstrated helped set the tone for those who would follow in the Section on General Social Service (later Section on General Service), formed in 1922.

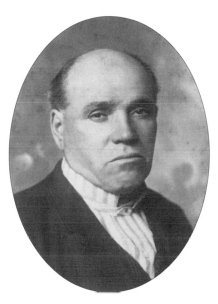

Jay Neville was an early live-in handyman for the Mayo family. A devoted, colorful figure, he later handled a variety of jobs in the Mayo's Masonic Temple offices.

Organization of General Service

Besides Jay Neville and Jack Craig, the early people involved in general service activities at Mayo included Cora Olson, who came in 1904, and William McDermott, who became doorman in 1910. Harry Harwick, former Clinic executive officer, credited Olson with setting the pattern for General Service philosophy at the Clinic, especially in her devotion to caring for patient needs.

Ronald A. Mitchell came to the Clinic to work in a variety of service tasks in the early 1920s. Later, his interest in medicine matured and he became a special student in dental surgery at Mayo before entering dental practice. During this same period, Edward Munson, an experienced ambulance man, came from the Twin Cities to meet the trains and shuttle patients between the Clinic and the hospitals. During the following years, ambulance duty became an important activity, and at one time included an 18-man team headed by Clarence Moehnke.

In May 1922, Rev. W. W. Bunge came to Mayo to help establish a General Service Bureau. This new section began the work of today's General Service. The section worked in close cooperation with the Section on Medical Social Service. Besides Bunge, the section's personnel included Anna Carr, Cora Olson, and Ronald Mitchell. Within a short time, the name of the section was shortened to General Service.

Since Bunge and his associates began General Service, many people have been associated with the section and its work. Besides Bunge, the section heads have been Harry Bennett, Clyde Crume, Robert Trusty, and today's James J. Chihak.

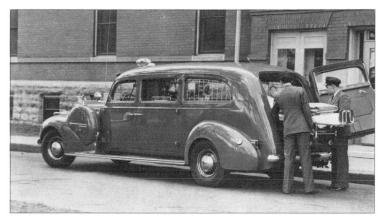

A General Service team prepares a Clinic ambulance for the next patient in 1940 — one of the many duties that personnel in this section have performed since its origins in 1922.

Medical Social Service

Social work at the Clinic began with Willa Murray, assisted by Cora Olson, in 1918. They were employed to help with the personal needs of the young women employed by Mayo. Patients soon discovered that their desks offered a place where information about rooms, hospitals, travel, etc., was available.

From these contacts, it became evident that there were patient needs for medical social service. In May 1921, Charlotte Bundy began the Section on Social Service in the Colonial Hospital. Isabella Gooding joined her shortly thereafter. As part of their varied activities, they helped institute a circulating hospital library program for patients. An occupational therapy program was initiated by volunteer workers.

In October 1922, the occupational therapy program was placed under the direction of Beatrice Hardy, a trained occupational therapy worker. The work was transferred to "The Little Green House" at 18 Second Avenue, Northwest, in 1925, where it remained until the building was removed in 1956 to make way for the new Rochester Methodist Hospital.

Elsie Eaton, a trained hospital librarian, was placed in charge of the circulating library program in 1923. She was followed by a series of librarians who worked with the Rochester Public Library in providing the books for distribution to patients.

The early medical social service section also arranged for interpreters to help international patients during their Clinic stay. Polish and Italian interpreters were regularly employed; people who spoke French, Greek, and Finnish were available as needed. The section supervised this activity until Gordon C. Harrison came in June 1951 to develop today's language department.

In February 1923, the offices of the Section on Social Service moved to Mayo Clinic. The same year, Charlene Buck, later Mrs. Herman J. Moersch, joined the staff. Buck's appointment established the commitment that all members of the section should be trained social workers.

In 1925, Bundy resigned her post as director of the medical social service program to become Mrs. James R. Learmonth, later Lady Learmonth. She was followed by Mrs. Helen Anderson Young. In 1927, Priscilla Keely, who joined the section in 1921, became director and remained so until 1953. Bundy and Keely thus became the major early contributors to the development of the present-day Medical Social Service. Since then, Evelyn Parkin (1953-1974), Judith A. Hayes (1975-1985), Vicki M. Duffney (1985-1990), and currently Michael W. O'Brien have headed the service.

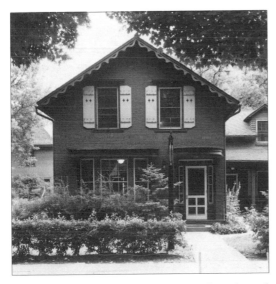

"The little green house" was the site of Mayo's occupational therapy program from 1925 to 1960.

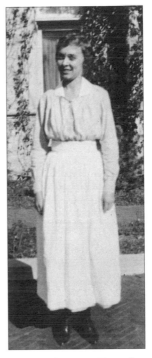

Charolette Bundy began Mayo's Social Service program in 1921.

147

Systems Section at Mayo

No matter what the period, visitors have often marveled at the organizational aspects of Mayo Clinic. From the first, the Mayo brothers were quick to adopt or introduce procedures that would ensure better efficiency in their practice. Dr. Henry S. Plummer helped develop systems and procedures for the collection, storage, and handling of medical records.

When Dr. Plummer was involved in planning the 1914 and 1928 Clinic buildings, he gave additional direction to the development of forms that reflected institutional needs. The establishment of a Coordinating Committee centralized much of the responsibility for this activity.

After World War II, it became evident that the growth of Mayo required a more systematic approach for procedural matters. This growth led, in 1947, to the formal organization of the Section on Procedures and Records (later, Systems and Procedures). Working with the Coordinating Committee, the first section head was Ernest H. Schlitgus. He had been with Mayo since 1928 and had been involved in the Clinic's desk system and registration department early in his career.

After a stint as director of the nonmedical personnel section, Schlitgus was tapped to head the new systems section. He remained section chief until 1964. During that period, many of Mayo's younger administrative assistants were assigned periodically to the section. It provided an excellent opportunity to learn about the daily procedural needs of Mayo.

Following Schlitgus, the section was headed by Richard W. Cleeremans. In recent years, he was followed by Craig A. Smoldt and currently Daniel E. Schaefer as head of the section.

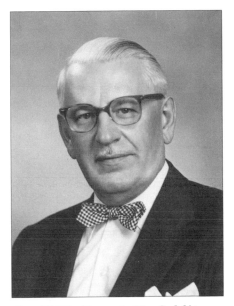

In 1947, Ernest H. Schlitgus became the first head of Mayo's Section on Procedures and Records (today's Systems and Procedures). Working with the Coordinating Committee, the new section helped refine and develop Clinic procedures.

Origins of Medical Illustrations and Photography at Mayo

The Mayo brothers recognized the value of the visual arts in medical science. Their talks and publications were often illustrated by drawings and photographs. Their employment of Dr. Louis B. Wilson in 1905 to develop Mayo's research laboratories hastened Mayo's use of the photographic process and medical illustrations.

Dr. Wilson's skills in photomicrography paved the way for the employment of Henry G. Andrews in 1907 to set up Mayo's first photographic laboratory at Saint Marys Hospital. Under Dr. Wilson's guidance, considerable skills were developed in photographing gross and microscopic specimens.

With the opening of the 1914 Building, the photographic studio transferred to new quarters there. In 1917, Andrews left Mayo and Earl Irish became head of Photography. He was followed in the leadership of the section by Leonard A. Julin, Stanley J. McComb, and James S. Martin.

Medical illustrations or graphics at Mayo traces its origins back to 1905, when an outside artist first did sketches of pathologic specimens. In 1907, Florence Byrnes was employed to handle this work under Maud Mellish Wilson's direction. Following Byrnes' marriage in 1909, Dorothy Peters took over the work until 1912, when Eleanora Fry was placed in charge.

Initially, the art studio was housed in the Clinic. In 1922, it moved to Saint Marys, and in 1959 was brought back to the Plummer Building. Following Eleanora Fry, Russell L. Drake, Vincent P. Destro, Robert C. Benassi, and currently, R. Michael Belknap have headed the section. Today's section combines medical illustration, photography, computer graphics, and graphic design.

Over the years, personnel in graphics and photography have been among the pioneers in developing their respective specialties. Today, members continue the search for excellence by employing the most modern computerized technology.

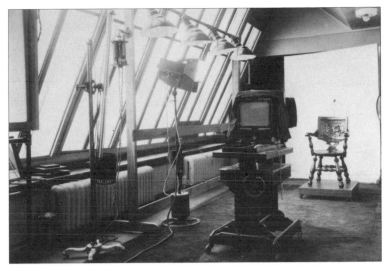

The Clinic photography studio before 1920. The activity had its beginnings in the work of Dr. Louis B. Wilson and Henry Andrews, around 1907, at Saint Marys Hospital.

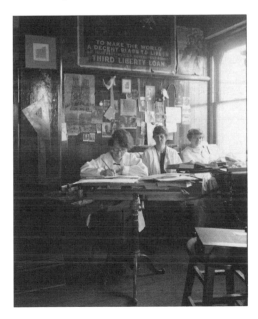

Members of the Mayo art studio at work around 1918. (Note the World War I patriotic poster.) They are, from left: Theodora Bergsland, Cora Olson, and studio head Eleanora Fry.

Correspondence at Mayo

In February 1909, Anna Edmondson, a native of Canada, came to Mayo as Dr. Charles H. Mayo's personal secretary. As a part of her duties, she began the organization and development of a division of correspondence for the growing practice. Until then, patient correspondence was handled by office assistants such as Alice Dodd and Cora Olson, who also had many other assignments.

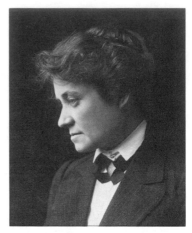

Anna Edmondson came to Mayo in 1909 as Dr. Charles Horace Mayo's personal secretary. She developed a division of correspondence for the growing firm. Upon her arrival, there were fewer than a dozen typewriters in use at the Clinic; 15 years later, there were nearly 200 machines.

Anna Edmondson began the correspondence work in a small room in the library building, which occupied the northeast corner of the present-day Plummer Building site. The work then transferred to a room adjoining the business office in the Masonic Temple. A year later, another move relocated it north of the Weber and Judd drugstore. With the opening of the 1914 Building, the correspondence division was again placed adjacent to the business office. Clinical space requirements, however, soon moved the division out of the 1914 Building to a more permanent home on the second floor of the business block located between the Zumbro Hotel and the Masonic Temple on First Avenue, Southwest. The correspondence work remained there for several decades.

In 1911, Frances Lind joined the division to help prepare correspondence for dictation. She later became the chief clerk in charge of the clerical section. In 1921, Lillian DeVilliers headed a new section in the division that handled the mail.

Continued growth of the Clinic soon made special secretaries necessary in the clinical and surgical sections. These people were responsible for the preparation of patient correspondence and the drafts of manuscripts written in a specific section. Edmondson developed a training program for these new secretarial positions. To assist their work, she also developed outlines of medical terminology.

When Edmondson arrived in 1901, there were fewer than a dozen typewriters in use throughout the Clinic. Fifteen years later, the number had grown to nearly 200. In 1923, Mr. C. L. Shandley joined the division's staff to handle typewriter repair and maintenance.

By 1926, the Correspondence Division had grown to employ some 69 people. They handled all the mail and telegrams for the Clinic, both incoming and outgoing. These people were also responsible for all the medical histories drawn from the Division of Records for correspondence purposes. Anna Edmondson remained active in the division until her retirement from Mayo in 1937. She died in 1959 in Canada.

"Joe Clinic"

For more than 45 years, Joseph Fritsch served Mayo in General Service. As the original door attendant of the 1928 Plummer Building until 1954, Fritsch became affectionately known by patients and Mayo people alike as "Joe Clinic."

His jovial, outgoing personality made him everyone's friend. He was often the first to meet patients as they entered the Clinic. People from all walks of life remembered his manner. At Christmas, he received many letters of thanks often just addressed to "Joe Clinic."

Born in England, Fritsch came to America with his parents as a school-age child. They finally settled in Rochester and Joe finished his schooling here.

In 1920, Fritsch became employed at the Clinic and later married another Clinic employee, Edna Mitchell. He retired from General Service in 1966 and died in Rochester 14 months later.

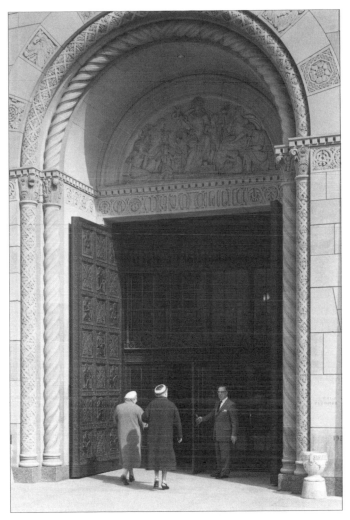

"Joe Clinic," as he became popularly known, greets people entering the Clinic. For 45 years, Joseph Fritsch was a familiar, friendly doorman for Mayo.

Christmas at Mayo

Historically, the yuletide season has always been a time for special get-togethers among Clinic personnel. After the erection of the 1914 Building, the main waiting room in the new structure became the setting for a number of Christmas gatherings for all the Clinic staff. Accounts of these events usually mention decorations, a tree, Santa Claus, and occasionally some form of entertainment or dancing. One announcement notes that "At 8:15 this evening (December 21, 1921), Father Christmas with his retinue of mummers, including Dr. Gardner as King of the Egyptians, his queen, and charming princess, will blaze the trail for his many followers."

It is difficult to date all of these earlier events, but between 1920 and 1925, they were held annually. After that period, sectional parties became commonplace until 1932. During that year, Dr. Boyd S. Gardner, head of the Dental Section, suggested that a general staff Christmas party would lift spirits during that bleak period in the Depression. His suggestion resulted in a three-year period of Christmas parties featuring local entertainment. The classic production in this series of get-togethers was the "75th Annual Convention of the Kombined Kick-A-Poo Kounty Medical Association," held on December 20, 1934. "President Wilburforce Airway" was in charge of the farce, which involved a number of locations in the 1914 Building for its proceedings. Folk remedies and patent cures were promoted during this delightful take-off on a medical meeting. The event concluded with a dance in the main floor waiting room.

After 1934, Christmas parties for all of the Clinic staff did not occur again until after the opening of Mayo Auditorium in 1938. The first of these occurred December 18, 1939, in the new facility, with Duke Ellington and his orchestra providing the dance music and assisting with preliminary entertainment. Ray Noble's band appeared the next year and Russ Morgan's group concluded the series in 1941. During the war years (1942-1944), no parties were held and the money saved was given to the USO and the county war chest for World War II.

Christmas parties for all of the Clinic staff were revived again in 1945, with Chuck Foster's band playing in Mayo Auditorium. He was followed by Charlie Spivak (1946), Wayne King (1947), Griff Williams (1948), Lawrence Welk (1949), Frankie Carle (1950), Lou Breese (1951), Jan Garber (1952), and Tony Pastor (1953).

In addition to these nationally known entertainment groups, several parties featured local entertainment and special productions. Two highlights were the "Folly of 1949" and the "Cosmorama of 1950." These locally produced productions ran as long as three hours, followed by a closing dance. As many as 200 Clinic people were involved, and two performances were required to accommodate all Clinic personnel. After 1953, it became apparent that the logistics of such get-togethers were impossible and the general Clinic Christmas party was discarded in favor of sectional gatherings.

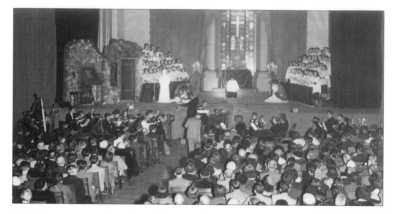

Christmas parties for all members of the Clinic family were popular during the 1920s and '30s. With Clinic growth following World War II, it became impossible to continue them. "Cosmorama of 1950" was one of the last shows to feature an extensive stage production, with some 200 people involved. Here is the "Christmas Fantasy" finale.

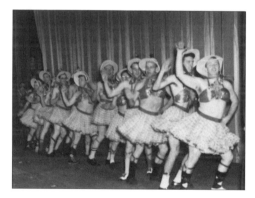

Christmas shows often included vaudevillian-style skits that spoofed daily life at the Clinic. The "Folly of 1949" featured the "Saddler Welles' Corpses de Ballet" — along with a stunning line of male dancers.

· SECTION IV ·

Mayo Office Facilities

In their early years, the Drs. Mayo used office space in several commercial buildings in Rochester. After the turn of the century, the Mayo brothers constructed some small structures for their sole occupancy, which adjoined their main offices in the Masonic Temple. These buildings were followed by the erection of the original Mayo Clinic Building in 1914. Under the visionary planning of Dr. Henry S. Plummer, this pioneering building became the model structure for Mayo's private group practice of medicine.

Siebens Building Historical Property

The Siebens Building occupies lots 7, 8, and 9 in Block 24 of Rochester's original plat. These three lots have been closely connected with Mayo's growth and development ever since William Worrall Mayo arrived in Rochester in 1863.

Initially, Block 24, which currently contains the Siebens and Plummer buildings on the west and the Kahler Plaza Hotel and the Centerplace Building on the east, was divided by an alley running east to west. Today, part of the vacated alley is used to link the Plummer and Siebens buildings and contains the massive bronze door entryway. Immediately north of this vacated alley is lot 7, which Dr. W. W. Mayo purchased on March 21, 1864, for $700 from Samuel H. and Cynthia Coon of Rochester. On this 40-by-140-foot lot, Charles Horace Mayo was born in 1865, in a small cottage.

On December 10, 1867, Dr. Mayo purchased lots 8 and 9, next to lot 7, for $100. Its sellers were Isaac W. and Charlotte E. Simonds of Rochester. This purchase made Dr. Mayo owner of the complete parcel on which the Siebens Building now stands. On June 19, 1868, he mortgaged all three lots to help fund additional improvements on the property. In time, an attractive victorian-style home was completed that was prominently featured in Minnesota's 1874 atlas.

For almost 50 years, the series of homes that were built on this land served the family in a variety of ways. At times, Dr. W. W. Mayo had his medical office there. To supplement family income, boarders and renters occupied rooms and homes on the site. The yard and outbuildings provided the Mayo brothers and sisters with space for youthful play. After Dr. Will's marriage in 1884 to Hattie Damon, the couple lived there and their first child, Carrie, was born there.

Around the turn of the century, 1900-04, the elder Mayo and his wife distributed their land holdings to their children. The Siebens site was given to their eldest daughter, Gertrude Berkman. In April 1912, Mrs. Berkman and her heirs conveyed the title to the Mayo brothers. The first Mayo Clinic building opened there on March 6,

160

1914, as a state-of-the-art facility.

During those early years, the property surrounding the site was essentially residential in character. With the erection of the impressive five-story Central School in 1868 across the street from the Mayo home, and the construction of a number of prominent churches on nearby corners, the Mayo property became strategically located, as it was between Rochester's cultural facilities and the growing commercial district immediately behind it.

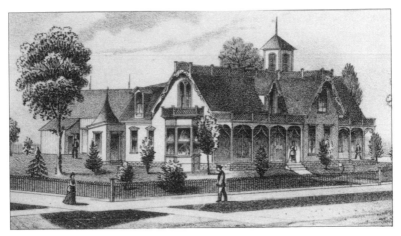

The residence of Dr. William Worrall Mayo as it appeared in the 1874 atlas of Minnesota. The home stood on the site of today's Harold W. Siebens Medical Education Building. Dr. Charles H. Mayo was born in an earlier home on the site .

Mayo and the Telephone

Mayo and its close attachment with communication devices has evolved from an event that occurred more than a hundred years ago.

According to family tradition, it was young Charlie Mayo who, at age 14, without benefit of instruction other than descriptions and pictures he had seen, put together the first telephone link in Rochester in 1879. The telephone connected Dr. W. W. Mayo's office and his farm residence in southeast Rochester. The installation was another example of mechanical dexterity that later aided Dr. Charlie in his accomplishments as an internationally renowned surgeon.

While the details of the phone incident are obscure, *The Record and Union* of Rochester makes reference to it in the following story from December 12, 1879:

The telephone line between Dr. Mayo's office and his residence is now up, the machines, or instruments, whichever they are, in position, and everything working splendidly. Conversation can be carried on just as rapidly and accurately as though the persons talking were only separated by a few feet instead of a mile, and familiar voices can be recognized as easily. Parties wishing to summon the Dr. between 6 (o'clock in the morning) and 9 (o'clock in the evening) can do so by making their wants known at Messrs. Geisinger and Newton's drug store. After 9 p.m. and before 6 a.m. it will be necessary to find Mr. George Tilsbury, the night watch, who will operate the instrument between the hours named when occasion demands. This will prove not only a convenience but a positive benefit to both the Dr. and his patients.

Interestingly, Dr. E. C. Cross, another Rochester physician, followed Dr. Mayo's lead two months later by stringing a telephone line between his home and office.

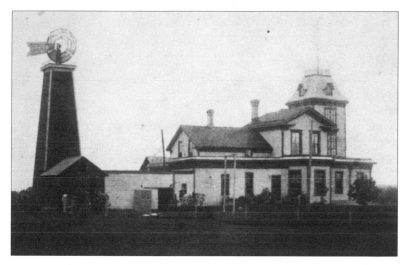

The Mayo farm in southeast Rochester was connected by a telephone link with Dr. William Worrall Mayo's downtown office in 1879. Tradition suggests that young Charlie made the hookups.

First Offices of the Drs. Mayo

On May 11, 1883, *The Record and Union* of Rochester reported:

Dr. Mayo has moved to his new rooms in the Cook block, opposite the post office. He has large reception and consulting rooms, and an operating room. All the rooms are light, airy and cheerful, and nicely furnished. There is no pleasanter office in the city. His son will return from Ann Arbor, Michigan, about the first of June and assist the Doctor in his extensive practice.

This newspaper story records the beginnings of the Mayo family partnership. The return of Dr. Will from medical school in 1883 launched the family group practice that later led to the development of Mayo Clinic.

The building where all this began still exists in Rochester. Over the years, it has been extensively remodeled and today houses Massey's department store. An historical plaque on the corner of the building notes its distinguished past.

As part of the Cook block, the structure was originally named the Ramsey Building. The Mayo offices were first located there over the drugstore of George Weber. During the 17 years that they occupied the building, the Mayos remodeled and expanded their offices many times. Eventually, they had rooms on both the ground floor and the upstairs. As their medical practice continued to grow, the Mayo firm finally relocated across the intersection to larger quarters in the new Masonic Temple Building on November 29, 1900.

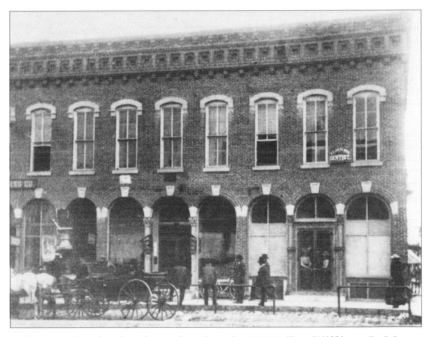

DR. WILLIAM W. MAYO, Hours 1:30 to 4 p. m.   Telephone No 252.
DR. WILLIAM J. MAYO, Hours 8 to 9 a. m., 1:30 to 4 p. m.   Telephone No. 112.
DR. CHARLES H. MAYO, Hours 8 to 9:30 a. m., 1:30 to 4 p. m.   Telephone 114.
DR. A. W. STINCHFIELD, Hours 8 to 9:30 a. m., 1:30 to 4 p. m.   Telephone 115.
DR. C. GRAHAM, Hours 11 a. m. to 12 m., 7 to 8 p. m.   Telephone 124.
Sunday Hours 11 a. m. to 1 p. m.
Office Corner Zumbro and Main Streets.   Telephone 211.

A business card produced around 1894 for the early Mayo offices in the Ramsey Building.

After medical school graduation in 1883, Dr. William J. Mayo joined his father in practice in this building (site of today's Massey's store). For 17 years, the Mayo partnership grew and flourished at this location before moving to the Masonic Temple in 1900.

Mayo Masonic Temple Offices

When the Masonic Temple Building was completed in January 1901, Drs. Mayo, Stinchfield, and Graham were already occupying their new offices in it. Located on the site of the present Centerplace Building, the three-story brick structure was 110 feet long by 50 feet wide. The first story provided space for Mayo offices and the Weber and Heintz drug store.

Until the completion of the first Clinic Building in 1914, the Masonic Building and its annexes housed the Mayo practice. The building was destroyed by fire in 1916. Another Masonic Building was erected in its place in 1917. In recent years, this structure was removed to make way for the present Centerplace Building.

Interestingly, three generations of the Mayo family played roles in the development of Masonry in Rochester. The father, William Worrall Mayo, became a Master Mason in 1863. His youngest son, Dr. Charlie, entered Masonry in 1890 and over the years was involved in the Knight Templars and the Shriners. He received a number of honors, including 33rd-degree Inspector General Honorary, Scottish Rite. Dr. Charlie's two sons, Drs. Charles W. Mayo and Joseph G. Mayo, were also active, with Charles W. Mayo receiving a variety of honors.

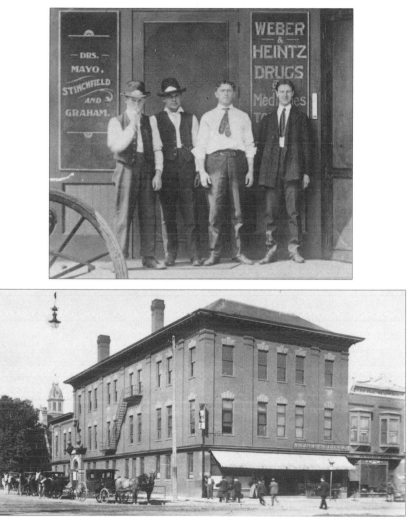

The Mayo brothers helped erect the Masonic Temple in 1900. They were among its first occupants. The Mayos expanded several times at this location, by constructing adjoining annexes, before they erected the 1914 Mayo Clinic Building.

1909 Mayo Library

One of the first buildings designed for and solely occupied by Mayo was the small, redbrick building that stood on the northeast corner of the 1928 Plummer Building location. Featuring a porch supported by four classically styled columns, the attractive two-story structure was set back from Second Street, Southwest. A well-kept floral garden grew in front of the building and further enhanced its appearance.

Erected in 1909, the structure provided space for Mayo's expanding publications division. Two years before, Maud H. Mellish had joined the Clinic to organize and develop a library and do editorial work. Mrs. Mellish, later Mrs. Louis B. Wilson, originally worked in Mayo's front office room of the old Masonic Temple. Within a short time, plans were drawn for the new building behind the temple.

When completed in 1909, the building's first floor featured a large room lined with cases for books; a circular, revolving reading table; and study tables. Staff meetings and lectures took place there. Two smaller rooms also were on the ground floor; one provided space for book stacks and the other offered space for editorial work.

The building's second floor had rooms for the art studio, coats, and storage. A corridor linked the facility with the Masonic Temple. Initially, ample space was available, but soon accommodations became cramped. The building continued to house publications until the completion of the 1914 Building. At that time, the division moved to the third floor of the new Clinic.

Afterwards, Dr. Melvin S. Henderson acquired the little building for the use of his Section on Orthopaedic Surgery. The section remained there until the structure was torn down to make way for the 1928 construction. At that time, the building's classic columns were salvaged for White Gables, the residence of Dr. and Mrs. (Edith Mayo) Fred W. Rankin, on Mayowood Road. The columns still grace the entryway of the home.

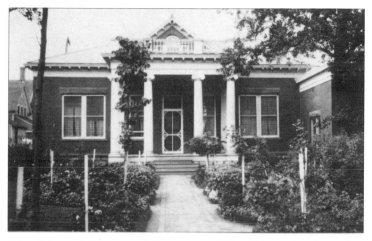

The Mayo Library, at the rear of the Masonic Temple, opened in 1909. Besides the medical library, the small structure housed an art studio. After the 1914 Clinic Building opened, the Section on Orthopaedics used the library before it was removed around 1926.

1914 Building Cornerstone Ceremonies

At 5 p.m. on Wednesday, October 9, 1912, members of the firm, Drs. Mayo, Graham, Plummer, and Judd, their associates, and other interested onlookers gathered on the southeast corner of Franklin (Second Avenue, Southwest) and Fourth Street (First Street, Southwest) to observe the cementing of the Missouri marble cornerstone into the wall of the first Mayo Clinic Building. It would be two more years before the structure would be completed, but the event was important in the evolution of Mayo's medical practice.

As part of the ceremonies, Dr. William J. Mayo said:

The object of this building is to furnish a permanent house wherein scientific investigation can be made into the cause of the diseases which afflict mankind, and wherein every effort shall be made to cure the sick and the suffering.

It is the hope of the founders of this building that in its use, the high ideals of the medical profession will always be maintained. Within its walls all classes of people, the poor as well as the rich, without regard to color or creed, shall be cared for without discrimination.

In these remarks, Dr. Will summarized the creed by which Mayo has been guided over the decades of its existence.

The conclusion of the brief cornerstone event was presided over by Dr. Charles H. Mayo. He initially spread the mortar over the stone. Drs. C. Graham, E. Starr Judd, and H. S. Plummer followed him in the task. In conclusion, Dr. Charlie placed in the stone a sealed copper-leaded box containing a miscellany of material relating to the day and the Mayo firm.

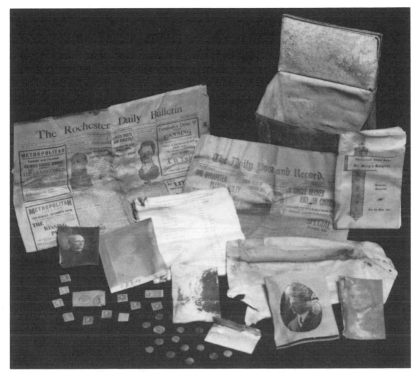

The cornerstone for the 1914 Mayo Clinic Building was laid on October 9, 1912. Dr. Charles H. Mayo officiated in spreading the mortar and installing a box of memorabilia. In 1986, the box was salvaged when the building was removed to allow the erection of the Siebens Building. Despite its wet condition, many items in the cornerstone box were saved — coins, stamps, newspapers, publications, and typewritten data.

Opening of 1914 Building

It was Friday, March 6, 1914, and some 1,600 people thronged to the opening of the new building of Drs. Mayo, Graham, Plummer, and Judd. Between the hours of 5-9 p.m., the Visiting Nurse Committee of the Civic League hosted the open house for the first Mayo Clinic Building. The small tour fee that they collected totaled nearly $400 by the evening's end. The funds helped maintain a visiting nurse in Rochester. Mrs. William J. Mayo and her 11 committee members helped direct the crowd. Fakler's orchestra provided background music for the event.

Members of the Mayo staff were stationed in the various departments of the building to give directions. Visitors used the right-hand or south stairway in going through the building's five floors. Return was by the left-hand or north stairway.

Constructed of reinforced concrete and finished with red Pennsylvania brick trimmed with Missouri marble, the building was designed by Ellerbe & Rounds of St. Paul. Mayo's planning committee consisted of Drs. Henry S. Plummer and Louis B. Wilson, along with Harry J. Harwick. Dr. Plummer was the driving force behind the structure and provided the architect with many insights into Mayo's unique needs.

Construction began in 1912. In addition to Ellerbe & Rounds, the following firms were involved: G. Schwartz & Co., the general contract; Maass & Co., the plumbing and heating; Linden Co. of Chicago, the decorating; Foster Electric Co., the electrical work; Rochester Telephone Co., the phone work; and F. J. Paine Co., the furniture.

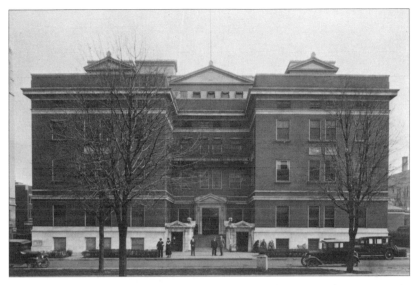

The original Mayo Clinic Building opened on March 6, 1914. A special open house was held with a modest charge to raise money for a visiting nurse in the city.

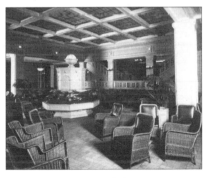

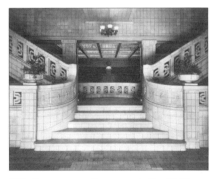

The spacious waiting room on the main floor of the 1914 Building was finished with attractive Rookwood tile on the floor and walls. A decorative fountain dominated the room.

Visitors to the 1914 Building open house used this attractive main staircase. It was made of architectural tile supplied by Rookwood Pottery, Cincinnati, Ohio.

Construction Details of 1914 Building

After the opening of the new Mayo Clinic Building in 1914, a number of stories regarding the structure appeared in the area press. Written in the florid style of that day, these reports are a major resource regarding the first Mayo Clinic Building.

The 1914 Building had engineering details that reflected that day's "cutting edge" technology. For example, near the double boilers (one for backup) in the basement, there was a large rotary valve vacuum cleaner. Stale air in the building was exhausted out of the top of the structure by a system of ventilating pipes. In cold weather, steam pipes warmed the fresh air being drawn into the building. A gas incinerator in the basement burned refuse. Nearby were coal bins that could accommodate 12 carloads. A pressure-controlling device regulated the city water entering the building.

In addition to these features, the new building incorporated an ingenious communications system that Dr. Henry S. Plummer had carefully devised. It has been called the first large intercommunicating telephone system in the United States. Using Dr. Plummer's specifications, the equipment allowed a physician to be paged and receive a telephone call anywhere in the building. By responding to a preassigned ticker code that was sounded throughout the building, the consultant could pick up a call at the most convenient phone available.

Coupled with the new telephone system, Dr. Plummer also devised a system of signal-lights in the corridors that helped identify the whereabouts of both physicians and patients. This replaced a simple mechanical signal system that had been used earlier.

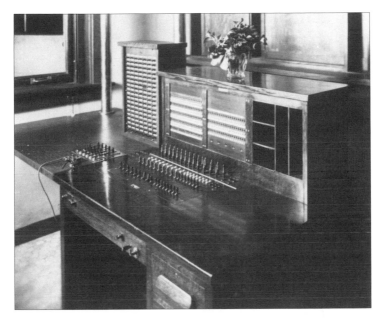

During the design of the 1914 Mayo Clinic Building, Dr. Henry S. Plummer and the architect, Ellerbe and Co., made easy communication a high priority. Operators used this telephone switchboard to page people throughout the building with a telegraphic code. The person being paged could pick up the call at several conveniently located points in the building. This has been called the first large intercommunicating system in the United States.

Construction of 1928 Building

Excavation for construction of the 1928 Plummer Building began in August 1926. The impressive steel skeleton was completed in May 1927. Laying of the exterior brickwork also started that month.

A brief cornerstone-laying ceremony was held for the partially finished building during the evening of June 22, 1927. Dr. Charles H. Mayo represented the Mayo brothers as Dr. Will was out of town. Dr. Charlie said:

Intelligence with knowledge enables wisdom to extend the highest service. Such service has made necessary this building which we now dedicate to the relief of suffering humanity through diagnosis, treatment, and cure of disease and the healing of wounds.

Dr. Henry S. Plummer and Harry Harwick also participated in the event.

During this stage of construction, the building plans did not include a tower large enough to house a carillon. A change in the plans was announced later in August 1927.

It was reported that the apex of the addition to house the carillon would be 55 feet above the present tower steelwork. The building's height was thereby increased to 295 feet, making the building the tallest in Minnesota at that time.

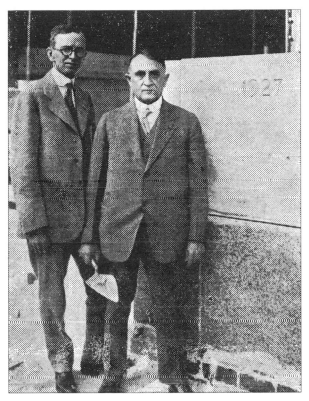

Drs. Charles H. Mayo (trowel in hand) and Henry S. Plummer help lay the cornerstone of the new Mayo Clinic Building (today's Plummer Building) on June 22, 1927. Dr. Charlie dedicated the structure to "the relief of suffering humanity through diagnosis, treatment, and cure of disease and the healing of wounds."

Rochester Carillon in Plummer Building

On Sunday, September 16, 1928, dedication ceremonies for the 23-bell Rochester Carillon were held on Second Avenue Southwest in front of the nearly completed Plummer Building. The street was blocked off to allow for the hour-long ceremony, which included performances by the Rochester Municipal Band, the Community Chorus, and the American Legion Drum Corps.

During the ceremonies, Dr. Will said:

Today, we dedicate this carillon to the American soldier, in grateful memory of heroic actions on land and sea to which America owes her liberty, peace, and prosperity.

The occasion culminated a plan proposed by Dr. Will many years before to construct a soldier's monument containing a bell tower. Several sites had previously been considered in Rochester, including College Hill. With the planning and construction of the 1928 building, it became evident that the height and architectural beauty of the structure resolved the question.

Interestingly, the carillon dedication served an additional purpose. In his remarks, Dr. Charlie mentioned the other:

. . . because of the great necessity of using the new Clinic Building as rapidly as the floors are completed, there will be no formal opening, and this day of dedication must serve. The Clinic is declared open.

Dr. Charlie further noted:

This building stands as a monument to the ability and genius of Dr. Henry S. Plummer, who has had full supervision of its design and erection, and he above all deserves credit for the detail and arrangement of its interior construction and arrangement of all the scientific and mechanical appliances which make accurate diagnosis not only possible but probable.

Originally, the bells of the carillon covered a range of two octaves. The largest of the 23 bells, or bass bell, weighs 7,840 pounds, with the total weight of the bells being 36,988 pounds. The original

178

bells came from the Gillett and Johnston Bell Foundry, Croydon, England.

In 1977, the descendants of Alphonso Gooding, a pioneer Rochester settler, extended the musical range of the carillon by presenting 33 bells varying in weight from 20 to 130 pounds. The new bells were cast at the Petit and Fritsen Bell Foundry, Aarle-Rixtel, Holland. This enlarged 56-bell carillon now has a range of four and one-half octaves.

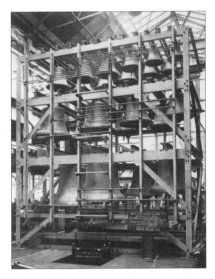

The Rochester Carillon in the Gillett and Johnston Bell Foundry, Croydon, England, before shipment to America in 1928. The 23-bell instrument featured a bass bell weighing 7,840 pounds.

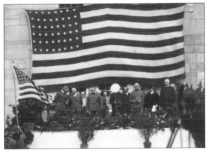

Dedication of the Rochester Carillon was held on September 16, 1928. The Mayo brothers wore military uniforms and the bells were dedicated to the memory of the American soldier.

Plummer Building Bronze Doors

On November 10, 1928, the solid bronze outer doors on the new Plummer Building were installed with the aid of a steam shovel. The two elaborately figured doors weigh 4,000 pounds each, stand 16 feet high, and are five and one-half inches thick. They were manufactured by the Flour City Ornamental Iron Company, Minneapolis, from drawings by the architect, Ellerbe & Company, St. Paul. The cost was about $12,000. The designs covering each of the door's surfaces complement the building's romanesque style. Ray Corwin, an Ellerbe employee, designed most of the sculpted ornamentation of the building, along with the bronze doors. Flour City employed Charles (Carlo) Brioschi to create model designs for the doors.

Both sides of the doors depict Minnesota life in alternating squares. The designs symbolize six Minnesota facets: education, the domestic arts, the mechanical arts, the fine arts, the sciences, and agriculture. Two other designs focus on Minnesota lore. Six related symbols are etched around each thematic square.

The doors were originally designed to be closed at the end of each Clinic day. They have remained open, though, only to be closed in ceremonial recognition of the passing of a prominent Mayo person. One exception was the 1963 assassination of President John F. Kennedy. Records are not clear about the exact number of closings. In addition to the Mayo brothers' funerals in 1939, information indicates the doors were closed for the funerals of Drs. Henry S. Plummer (1936), Donald C. Balfour, Sr. (1963), Charles W. Mayo (1968) and Harry J. Harwick (1978). There is speculation, however, that other Mayo persons were honored: among those may have been Drs. E. Starr Judd and Joseph G. Mayo.

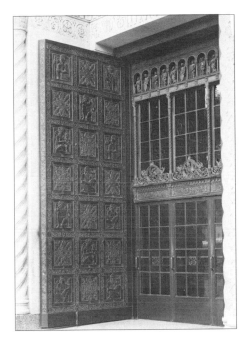

The solid bronze doors of the Plummer Building were installed on November 10, 1928. Weighing 4,000 pounds each, they stand 16 feet high and are five and one-half inches thick.

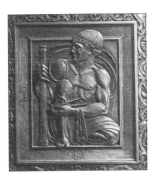

Decorative squares, which are repeated several times on the Plummer Building bronze doors, symbolize six Minnesota themes: education, domestic arts, mechanical arts, fine arts, science, and agriculture.

Plummer Building Exterior

People often enjoy viewing the varied decorations of Mayo's 1928 Plummer Building. While the building's romanesque style is evident, its exterior is also sprinkled with mythological and allegorical themes of a different origin.

The Bedford stone (Indiana limestone) that covers the outside of the building's two lower floors contains a series of carvings that focus on a variety of subjects relating to medicine, America, Minnesota, and Rochester. Of particular interest are carvings that reflect the times and locale of the building.

On the building's lower exterior, facing Second Avenue, Southwest, there are depicted: a bird, an eagle, a rabbit, a buffalo, a squirrel, fish, a Viking ship (part of Minnesota's heritage), St. George slaying a dragon (patron saint of England, birthplace of Dr. William Worrall Mayo), a pelican in its nest, a trimotored airplane (the type that first landed at Rochester), and a cartoon of Dr. H. S. Plummer examining the building's plans.

The side of the building that faces Second Street, Southwest, includes the following: a motorboat on a Minnesota lake, a partridge, flying geese, two gophers, three parrots, a swan, the insignia of Minnesota, the skull of an ox, a ram, the United States insignia, and a wildcat.

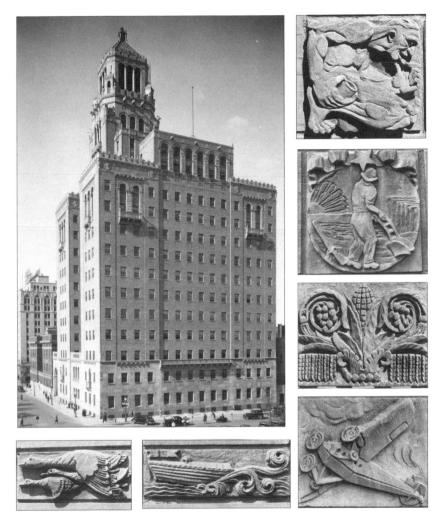

The Plummer Building's lower two floors are covered with Bedford stone (Indiana limestone). Scattered among the limestone are decorative carvings whose themes reflect medicine, America, Minnesota, and Rochester.

Memento of 1928 Presidential Race

The outcome of a national election is graphically recorded among the ornamental cartoons in stone that are scattered along the lower exterior base of Mayo's 1928 Plummer Building. While the depictions generally represent some aspect of Minnesota life, two special stones reflect the outcome of the 1928 presidential campaign.

During that period, Herbert Hoover ran for the presidency of the United States under the Republican banner. Al Smith opposed him as the Democratic candidate. Dr. Henry S. Plummer, Mayo representative on the new Clinic building construction, was a staunch supporter of the Republican cause, and John J. Raskob, a close, admired friend, was the National Democratic campaign manager. During the electioneering, the men enjoyed friendly exchanges concerning the merits of each other's candidate.

In November 1928, Hoover won the presidential race over Smith. The victory provided workers on the Clinic building with an opportunity to enliven the surface detail of the new building's lower floors. With Dr. Plummer's approval, two decorative stones were carved that depict the national party symbols in poses symbolic of the election's outcome.

One stone carving features a triumphant Republican elephant with its head elevated. Another carving depicts a dejected Democratic donkey with its ears drooping and its tail between its legs. The two stones are an interesting and unusual sight among the dozen or so carvings that are scattered nearby on the building's southern exterior.

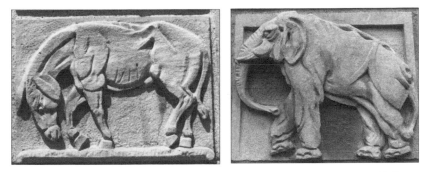

Two carvings on the lower south side of the Plummer Building reflect the 1928 presidential race. The dejected donkey symbolizes the defeated Democratic contender, Al Smith. The triumphant elephant symbolizes the successful Republican candidate, Herbert Hoover.

Franklin Station

Since 1928, the operations of Mayo's medical center in downtown Rochester have been lighted, heated, and cooled by the output of the Franklin Station. Jointly owned by Mayo and the Kahler Corporation, construction of the facility began in 1926 and was completed in 1928. It was designed to supply electric power, heating steam, process steam, cold well water, and hot softened water to its owners' buildings.

Dr. Henry S. Plummer played a prominent role in the plant's original planning. Ellerbe & Company was the architect. The building was planned to handle the new 1928 Clinic building and the adjoining Kahler properties, including several downtown hospitals.

The original equipment consisted of three 35,000-pound-per-hour boilers, two 1,000-kilowatt double-extraction turbo generators, two deep wells, three water softeners, and the instruments required to operate them. Over the years, the plant has been updated to meet the needs of its owners. Between 1950-1952, a six-story addition was built to the south of the original structure to house refrigeration equipment to cool the Mayo and Kahler buildings. Since then, improvements have met the needs of Mayo's expanded campus.

Coal initially was used to operate the plant. (The inside of an early boiler once provided dining space for some 26 members of a visiting engineering group.)

At the urging of Dr. H. S. Plummer, natural gas was brought to Rochester and the plant converted to accommodate its use in 1932. In January of that year, the plant became the first to receive natural gas in Minnesota. Shortly afterwards, the Rochester municipal power plant became the first municipally owned plant in the state to receive natural gas. In recent years, the Franklin Station has used gas and fuel oil on an alternating basis.

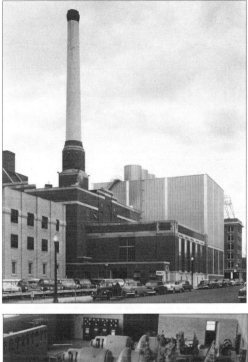

In 1928, Mayo Clinic and the Kahler Corporation jointly built the Franklin Station to supply lights, heat and, over time, refrigeration for their adjacent buildings. Dr. Henry S. Plummer had a significant role in planning the facility.

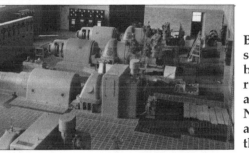

Between 1950 and 1952, a six-story addition was built to help house refrigeration equipment at the Franklin Station. New generators were also installed to improve the Franklin's capacity.

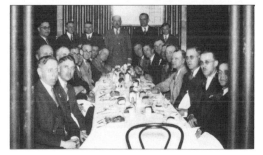

The Franklin station was initially operated by coal. In 1926, 26 members of a Minnesota engineering society dined in one of the newly built boilers.

187

Medical Sciences Building

In 1941, the original part of the Medical Sciences Building opened to provide additional facilities for laboratory research. The main research laboratories of the Clinic had been housed about three miles southwest of Rochester in the Institute of Experimental Medicine. The new science building later became the northern third of the present-day Medical Sciences Building. The original building has undergone two expansions since its erection.

In 1942, a small aeromedical unit was added to the south of the original structure. It featured a human centrifuge, pressure chambers, and a cold chamber. During World War II, the work of this unit was classified and off-limits to regular Clinic activities.

Construction on the last major addition to the Medical Sciences Building began in 1949. This addition, immediately south of the original structure, completely surrounded the aeromedical unit and more than doubled the size of the original structure. Remodeling of the older structure made it an effective part of the completed Medical Sciences Building. Dedicated in 1952, the expanded Medical Sciences Building was a model in laboratory sophistication.

The building featured Frank C. Mann Hall, an auditorium seating 180 people; a heart catheterization room; a human centrifuge; an engineering shop; pressure chambers; controlled temperature rooms; a mass spectrometer; radioactive isotope rooms; and other rooms for Anatomy, Biochemical Research, Biophysics, Electroencephalography, Physiology, and Surgical Research.

On September 26, 1952, Vannevar Bush, of the Carnegie Institution, spoke at the dedicatory ceremonies. Since then, the Medical Sciences Building has played an important role in Mayo's research activities.

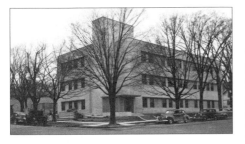

The first part of the Medical Sciences Building opened in 1941. Two additions in 1942 and 1952 increased the building's footage to its present size.

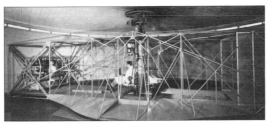

Dr. Earl H. Wood, center, seated at the controls of Mayo's human centrifuge in the aeromedical addition, located immediately south of the original Medical Sciences Building, in 1942. The classified studies, undertaken on the Mayo centrifuge by a team of investigators, produced fundamental knowledge that led to the production of anti-gravity or "G" suits for World War II fighter pilots.

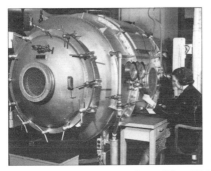

Technician Lucille Cronin at the controls of a pressure chamber in the aeromedical addition to the Medical Sciences Building. The chambers were used for classified studies during World War II. Researchers used Mayo's BLB oxygen mask to determine human oxygen requirements at various simulated altitudes. The work produced a series of high-altitude oxygen masks. The U.S. military used great numbers of these masks during and after the war to protect pilots from oxygen deficiencies.

Homestead Village and the Harwick Building

Two major building projects started at Mayo in the early 1960s. On May 31, 1960, groundbreaking was held for the Homestead Village development in southeast Rochester. The 102-unit project replaced the prefabricated Quonsets erected by Mayo after World War II in the Graham Addition to house residents of Mayo Graduate School of Medicine. The new Homestead Village featured 17 two-story, six-apartment buildings erected between Mayo's Homestead Addition and the Southgate Shopping Center. Ellerbe & Company of St. Paul was the architectural firm for the development.

Construction of Mayo's second 1960 building project began in August. Initially described as the "Biometrics Building," the new structure was designed to provide much-needed storage space for Mayo's valuable file of medical records and X-rays.

The structure was named the Harwick Building after Mayo's pioneer administrator, Harry J. Harwick. It featured three stories above the ground and a subway level for X-ray storage. After its occupancy in 1961, a vertical addition was announced in 1964. It provided four more floors above the original structure to house the offices of the Division of Education, the Computer Center, and the Section of Medical Statistics and Epidemiology.

The present-day Harwick Building is the result of another expansion in 1978-80 that provided additional administrative space. Ellerbe & Company, St. Paul, supplied architectural services for the first two stages of the building's construction. Harry Weese Associates, Chicago, provided the expanded design for the current Harwick Building.

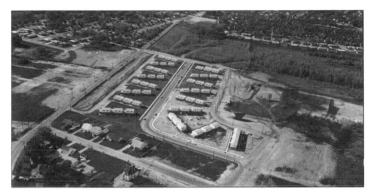

Homestead Village was constructed in southeast Rochester in 1960. The development featured 17 two-story, six-apartment buildings to house residents and their families.

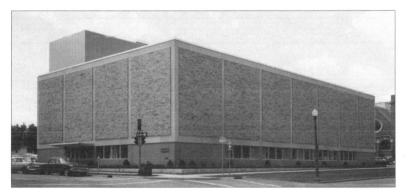

The original part of the Harwick Building opened in 1961. It was named after Harry J. Harwick, pioneer Mayo administrator. The building was expanded in 1964 and again between 1978 and 1980.

The Mayo Building

In early 1955, the Mayo Building was completed. Construction of the 10-story diagnostic facility had begun in 1950. It was the largest building project undertaken by Mayo up to that time. The overall size of the structure was equivalent to a 1,150-room office building.

After World War II, the number of patients who sought medical treatment at Mayo increased sharply. Studies from 1938 through 1949 showed that, each year, between 25,000 and 50,000 patients could not obtain appointments at Mayo because of the high demand for services. Under these circumstances, the construction of a new building was approved.

Ellerbe & Company was architect for the new facility. Working closely with several Clinic committees, designers carefully reviewed the operational system used in the older Clinic building. As a result of these studies, they conceived a building design that offered convenience and comfort for patients and residents of Mayo Graduate School of Medicine. The design featured systems for the efficient scheduling and routing of patients, physicians, and medical records, and a physical layout for convenient consultation among members of the medical staff.

The new building was constructed in the shape of a Greek cross. A typical floor housed eight sections of internal medicine, each of which included 11 examining rooms, a consultation room, a staff room, a secretarial office, and a seminar room for graduate medical programs and conferences. A central waiting room served two reception desks. The two appointment desks that were assigned to each reception desk handled two medical sections arranged along two corridors. Behind each reception desk was a file and clerical area for the four medical sections served by that desk. A system of chutes and conveyers expedited the movement of histories and other information to the various floors. Fifteen elevators allowed convenient access to all floors of the building for both patients and staff.

The bolted steel frame with concrete fireproofing around

192

columns and beams was reinforced to accommodate future expansion. The exterior of the building was covered with white and gray Georgia marble and trimmed with a gray aluminum. A mixture of marble from Italy, Portugal, and the United States decorated the main floor. Various types of wood finished the rooms on the upper floors. In an innovative decorative art program using the theme "Mirror to Man," a series of murals covered one complete wall of the central waiting room on each floor.

In 1966, an eight-floor expansion of the building was initiated. Completed in 1970, the addition increased the height of the building to almost 300 feet. Recently, a large telecommunications dish was installed on the structure's roof to receive satellite transmissions from Mayo's facilities in Jacksonville, Florida, and Scottsdale, Arizona.

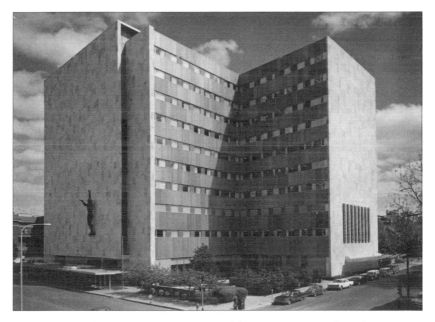

The original ten-story Mayo Building was completed in 1955. Construction began in 1950. Its size was equivalent to a 1,150-room office building. An eight-story addition, constructed between 1966 and 1970, brought its height to almost 300 feet.

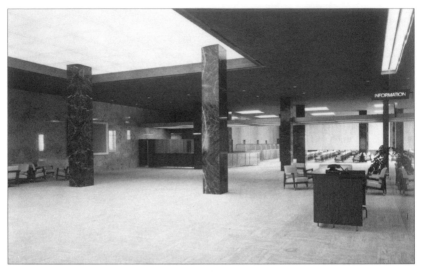

The main lobby of the Mayo Building at the time of its opening in 1955. It has been extensively remodeled since then.

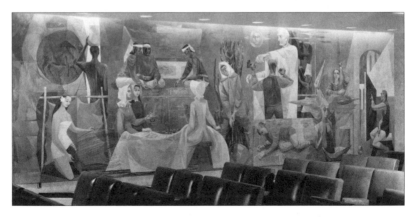

As part of the "Mirror to Man" art program in the new Mayo Building, thematic murals were commissioned for each of the building's central waiting rooms. This mural is located on the fourth floor and is entitled "Man and the Art Form."

· SECTION V ·
Mayo Hospital Facilities

The Mayos originally cared for local patients in private homes. In the case of out-of-town patients, the Mayos provided surgical treatment and aftercare in hotels and rooming houses in the city. With the opening of Saint Marys Hospital in 1889, Mayo patients received a dedicated hospital service. In the 1910s, the Kahler Corporation developed additional hospital facilities for Mayo's growing practice. Rochester Methodist Hospital acquired the Kahler hospital properties in 1954 and opened its present structure in 1966.

Early Mayo Surgery at the Carpenter House

As the surgical skills of Dr. William Worrall Mayo attracted more out-of-town patients to Rochester, he began using rooms at the American House, the Merchants Hotel, and the Norton Hotel to perform his operative procedures. After his eldest son, Dr. Will, joined him in 1883, it became customary for them to use the Norton Hotel and then the Carpenter House for operations on transient patients.

Located at 621 North Broadway, the Carpenter House was the first home of the Mayos' surgical clinics. Mrs. Caroline V. Carpenter and her family lived there. She was a capable practical nurse who was willing to make rooms available for nursing care. Her home could accommodate eight or nine patients at a time.

Initially, local physicians gathered at the Carpenters' to watch Dr. Mayo's major operations. In time, physicians from nearby towns were notified of important forthcoming operations. These were scheduled on Sunday mornings so those coming could more easily drive to Rochester. On these occasions, Dr. Mayo answered the visitors' questions and explained the procedure.

Also, late in 1888, the Carpenter House became the scene of young Dr. Will's first operation for a large ovarian tumor. The procedure was originally scheduled for his father, but the elder Mayo was delayed in returning to Rochester. Dr. Will stepped in and successfully removed a tumor that completely filled a washtub.

At Mrs. Carpenter's, the Mayos used a portable table and an operating set-up they could move from room to room. The home had no separate operating facility, though one room on each of the dwelling's two floors seems to have been favored.

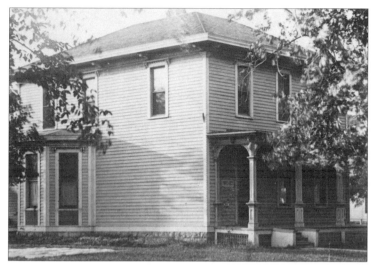

Dr. William Worrall Mayo used the Carpenter House at 621 North Broadway for many of his out-of-town surgical cases between 1883 and 1889. Caroline V. Carpenter was a capable practical nurse who made rooms available for medical care. The Mayos' surgical clinics for area physicians took place in the house. The Mayos later acknowledged that experience gained at the Carpenter House aided them in planning Saint Marys Hospital.

1883 Tornado

Despite their negative effects, natural disasters can stimulate public awareness and often dramatize community needs. This was the case early in the development of Mayo Medical Center in Rochester, Minnesota. In 1883, a tornado (then called a cyclone) created a major local emergency that brought together the Drs. Mayo and the Sisters of Saint Francis, a Catholic charitable order, in a community-wide effort to care for victims of the storm.

The summer of 1883 had been typical for midwestern America. Unstable air masses had formed over the region's broad plains and produced intermittent storms dotted with deadly twisters whose toll in lives and property created a variety of community emergencies. Olmsted County in southeastern Minnesota and its county seat of Rochester were among the few areas to suffer, within a month's time, the effects of two tornadoes.

On July 21, 1883, a twister raced through the rural areas of Olmsted County, just missing the city of Rochester. An eastbound passenger train was caught in its path and blown over, and 25 people were injured. Nearby Elgin was almost destroyed, and most of its 250 residents were affected. The storm caused only two deaths.

A month later, on August 21, 1883, Olmsted County was visited again by another, more devastating, tornado. Occurring in the evening hours, it caused destruction first in Dodge County, west of Olmsted, where five persons were killed. The storm entered Olmsted County through two rural townships and caused extensive farm damage. Around 7 p.m. the full fury of the tornado hit Rochester. Damage in the business district was spotty, but the pioneer residential area, around and north of the railway tracks west of Broadway, received the full effect of the twister. Called Lower Town, its houses and animals were literally swept away.

The storm exited Rochester by a northeasterly path through several townships, where it continued to produce heavy farm damage. One summary stated that Olmsted County residents suffered 31 deaths and 50 serious injuries.

At the end of the storm, relief forces quickly organized. At 8:30

a.m. the next day, Samuel Whitten, the mayor of Rochester, appointed a committee to deal with relief measures. Rommel Hall was made an emergency hospital, and 34 patients were brought there for further care. Dr. David M. Berkman, the son-in-law of Dr. William W. Mayo, was appointed hospital steward.

In the city, emergency help extended to some 233 families and 101 men. The Rochester committee eventually arranged the building of 51 houses, and 15 dwellings were built privately. Some 106 families received assistance in other rebuilding. More than 255 families received bedding, and some 570 persons were provided with clothing. Relief money came into the city from as far away as Chicago. At the end of three months, the relief committee reported receipts of $69,577.25 along with provisions amounting to $45,716. Among the generous contributors were many churches.

Years later, Dr. William W. Mayo, father of the Mayo brothers, recalled how the Sisters of Saint Francis assisted in the crisis. He told how Mother Alfred Moes, founder and leader of the Catholic teaching order, prevailed on him afterward to help plan a community hospital.

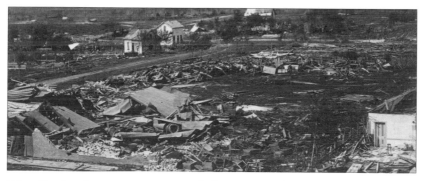

The Rochester area was struck by two major "cyclones" in the summer of 1883. While the first passed north of town, the second hit the pioneer section of Rochester on the evening of August 21, 1883. It left a trail of death and destruction that prompted an outpouring of relief efforts. The Sisters of Saint Francis and the Drs. Mayo played leading roles in caring for the injured.

Saint Marys Hospital

On September 30, 1889, Dr. Charles H. Mayo performed what may have been the first surgical procedure at the newly constructed Saint Marys Hospital. He was assisted by his brother, Dr. William J. Mayo, and his father, Dr. William W. Mayo, who administered the anesthetic agent. The operation was for removal of a cancerous growth of the eye.

Although the hospital had been scheduled to accept patients on October 1, 1889, the facility was ready and the Mayos decided to undertake the surgical procedure a day early. Recently discovered information suggests that this case was not the hospital's first patient. Regardless of who was first and when, we do know that patients were admitted to the new facility some weeks before the dedication of the building in October. The hospital has been in continuous operation ever since.

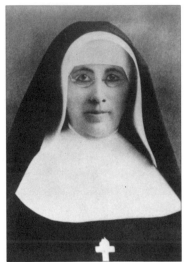

Mother Alfred Moes was the driving force behind the formation of Saint Marys Hospital. She prevailed upon Dr. William Worrall Mayo to assist in its planning after the 1883 tornado. By frugal living, the Sisters of Saint Francis raised funds to purchase the property and begin construction.

The devastating tornado that hit Rochester on August 21, 1883, provided the impetus for establishing the hospital. After this tragic event, the Sisters of Saint Francis, a Catholic charitable teaching order, helped care for the injured and homeless. During that time, Mother Alfred Moes, leader of the order, observed that Rochester seemed to need a hospital. When the emergency was over, Mother Alfred approached her friend Dr. William W. Mayo with her idea about establishing a hospital in the city. He did not initially think that the project was feasible. After she persisted, however, he agreed to help her plan the facility, provided funds could be obtained.

Some four years of hard work, frugal living, and saving followed, and the Sisters finally were able to purchase nine acres of land for the new facility in 1887 at a cost of $2,200. The acreage was located west of the city limits. After assembling plans and suggestions from the Mayos, Mother Alfred initiated contracts for the new project in August 1888.

The three-story structure was constructed of red brick, with window ledges of white, rough-hewn stone. The main floor featured a reception area, doctors' offices, dining facilities, and a kitchen. On the second floor, a 12-foot-square operating room was installed. A bay of three windows topped by a large skylight dominated the exterior wall, filling the room with a soft northerly light.

The floor was inclined slightly, so cleaning solutions could drain into a waste pipe. Prominent among the room's equipment was an operating table that Dr. Charlie had constructed. Private rooms and women's wards completed the floor. A men's ward, chapel, and recreation room were located on the third floor. The total capacity of the facility was 27 beds. The new hospital was open to all patients, regardless of religion, sex, race, or economic circumstances.

Since then, Saint Marys Hospital has grown to accommodate some 1,100 beds, and along with Rochester Methodist Hospital, it continues to provide care for all hospital patients at Mayo Clinic in Rochester.

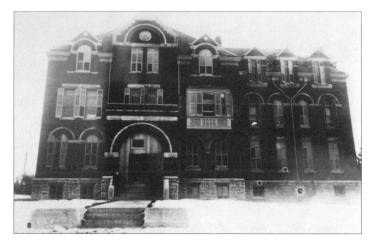

At its opening, Saint Marys Hospital had a 27-bed capacity. It was open to all classes of patients. According to tradition, Dr. Charles H. Mayo performed the first surgical procedure there on September 30, 1889. (Courtesy Saint Marys Hospital.)

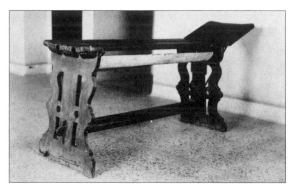

Dr. Charles H. Mayo built the first operating room table for Saint Marys Hospital. It featured an adjustable headrest and was the main fixture in the original 12-foot-square operating room. (Courtesy Saint Marys Hospital.)

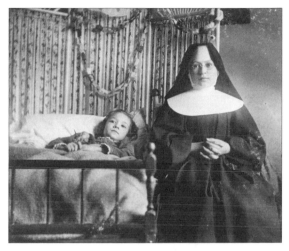

One of the Sisters of Saint Francis caring for a young child at the hospital around 1898. Decorations were made to enliven the patient's room and provide a symbol of friendship.

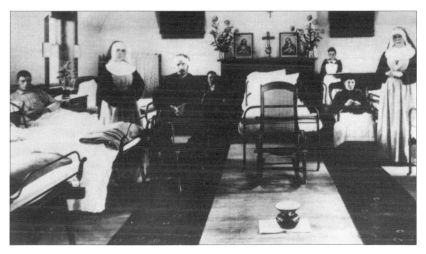

A ten-bed ward at Saint Marys Hospital around 1889. The spittoon in the center was conveniently located for patients to use.

Chute Sanitarium

Shortly after the turn of the century, Charles H. Chute and his wife, Margaret, converted their boardinghouse into a sanitarium. Located near the railroad tracks at 117-123 Third Street, Northwest, the Chute Sanitarium quickly became a popular place for patients from the rural area.

One source indicates that the sanitarium had a 15-bed capacity when it opened in 1906. Over the next three years, the popularity of the facility encouraged its proprietors to erect a number of additions. By 1909, the three-story frame building facing Central Park could handle 90 beds and included a small operating room. Along with the Cook Hotel, it was used for the early surgical cases assigned to Mayo's new orthopedic section. Among the Clinic surgeons who operated there were Drs. Judd, Beckman, Henderson, and Meyerding. Initially, Millie Hanson supervised several practical nurses. The charges were $1 a day for a ward bed and $1.50 for a single room. Board was included.

In 1916, the Chute Sanitarium discontinued operations, and the building was converted into the Watson Hotel. Before its removal, it functioned as the Parkside Hotel.

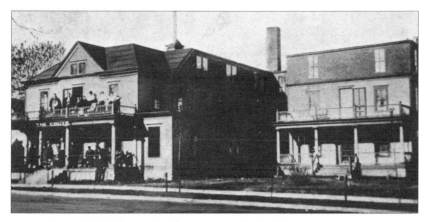

Charles H. Chute and his wife, Margaret, converted their boardinghouse into the Chute Sanitarium around 1906. Located near the railroad, the Chute became popular with rural patients. Drs. E. S. Judd, M. S. Henderson and E. H. Beckman operated there.

Kahler Hotel

By 1906, there was such need for additional hospital space in Rochester that John H. Kahler, manager of the Cook Hotel, formed a company to provide additional hospital facilities for the Clinic. Initially, the residence of E. A. Knowlton was purchased by Kahler's newly formed Rochester Sanatorium Company, a forerunner of the Kahler Corporation.

The Knowlton home stood on the corner of Second Avenue, Southwest and Center Street (present Damon Building block). After its purchase, an extensive brick addition was constructed, and the first Kahler Hotel, or Sanatorium as it was also called, opened to the public on May 4, 1907. It featured the new concept of the convalescent hotel with a hospital unit and surgical facilities available on its third floor. The success of the new venture soon led to the erection of another addition in 1909.

Over the next decade, John Kahler and several other businessmen in Rochester erected a number of such dual-purpose facilities. Among these was the Zumbro Hotel, which had an operating room when it opened in 1912.

The present Kahler Hotel opened on September 27, 1921. It featured 210 hospital beds, 150 beds for convalescent patients, and 220 beds for general hotel purposes. Three operating rooms were located where the Penthouse restaurant is today.

At that time, the original Kahler was renamed the Damon Hotel in honor of Mrs. William J. Mayo's father. The Damon name was carried over to the Clinic building that now occupies the former Damon Hotel block.

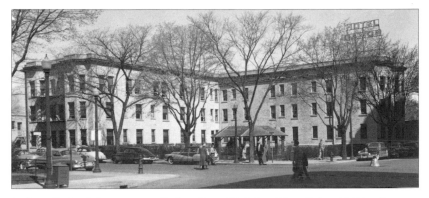

John H. Kahler opened the first Kahler Hotel in 1907. It was renamed the Damon Hotel after the opening of the present Kahler Hotel in 1921. The Damon name came from the family of Dr. Will's wife.

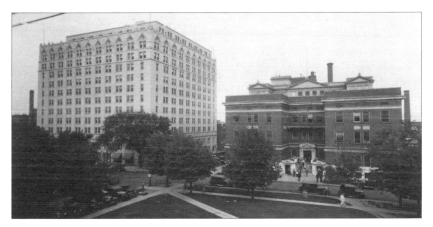

The first building of today's Kahler Hotel opened in 1921 across from the 1914 Mayo Clinic Building. Its upper floors were used as a hospital, the middle floors were for convalescent care, and the lower floors for hotel guests.

Zumbro Hotel

A year before work began on the Clinic's first building, ground was broken in downtown Rochester for one of the city's most imposing construction projects. In the spring of 1911, the Zumbro Hotel Company began construction of a new $150,000 hotel which would "surpass anything of the kind in this portion of the state." Initially planned to be four stories in height, its construction continued upward for another story after John H. (Jack) Kahler, company president, wired a request while on a trip to Europe.

When it opened on March 9, 1912, the Zumbro Hotel was the tallest building in the city. The "enchanting garden view" from atop the structure offered "a picture no artist could paint." The facility featured 122 bedrooms, 65 baths, nine sample rooms for commercial men, a barber shop, and a pool room. However, the demand at Mayo for hospital beds was so great that 48 of the Zumbro rooms were immediately assigned for hospital patients and an operating room. This arrangement continued until March 1915.

As the hotel needs continued to grow, the small, older West Hotel immediately behind the Zumbro was removed, and an eight-story annex to the Zumbro opened in 1917. Mayo soon enlisted the new annex to meet its space needs. Mayo rented floor after floor of the Zumbro Annex to house medical offices and laboratories. Finally, only the first and top floors of the Zumbro Annex remained for hotel purposes. To facilitate Mayo access, the annex was linked with the original Clinic building by Rochester's first skyway over the alley separating them. With the opening of the 1928 building, Mayo's occupancy of the structure changed.

The Zumbro Hotel was an important step in the development of the present-day Kahler Corporation, which was formed in 1917. Like other properties, services at the Zumbro Hotel changed to meet the needs of each generation. For example, during one period it was a favorite hotel for the many Spanish-speaking people who came to the Clinic. In September 1987, it was demolished and the Kahler Plaza Hotel erected in its place.

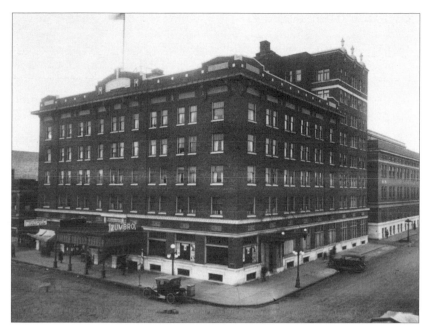

The Zumbro Hotel opened in 1912 on the site of today's Kahler Plaza Hotel. It was the tallest building in the city and had 122 beds. Mayo Clinic immediately used 48 beds for hospital patients.

Colonial Hospital

In March 1915, the Colonial Hotel-Hospital opened in Rochester. Its original capacity was 175 beds with two operating rooms for minor procedures and emergencies. Within two years, the hospital needs of Mayo patients required use of the whole structure, and the hotel operation ended.

In 1916, a wing to the south of the original building was completed. A year later, the hospital's capacity increased to 244 beds with the addition of another floor to the building's central wing, which also provided four new operating rooms. In the early 1930s, another floor was added to the other two wings and, in 1949, the north wing was completed, giving the building its final look.

Originally constructed by Roberts Hotel Company, the Colonial became part of Kahler-Roberts Corporation in 1917. The Colonial Hospital remained an important part of the Kahler Corporation until the newly formed Rochester Methodist Hospital acquired it, along with the Worrall Hospitals, in 1954. Since then, the newer wing of the building has housed many Rochester Methodist Hospital activities.

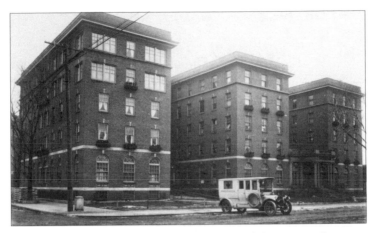

The Colonial Hotel-Hospital opened in 1915. It soon became all-hospital and a third wing was added in 1916. The fourth wing was completed in 1949.

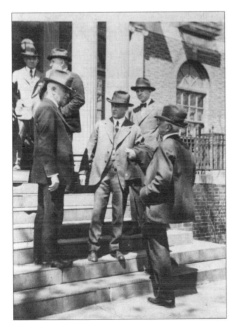

The Mayo brothers, Dr. Will (left) and Dr. Charlie (center), along with John Kahler (right), made regular checks of the Colonial Hospital and other Kahler hospitals in downtown Rochester.

Worrall Hospital and Annex

The Worrall Hospital was opened by the Kahler Corporation in January 1919. The new Mayo-affiliated facility was named in honor of Dr. William Worrall Mayo, the Mayo brothers' father, and was located at 215 Third Street, Southwest, on the site of today's Hilton and Guggenheim buildings.

The hospital contained five operating rooms for the surgical specialties of ophthalmology, otolaryngology, rhinology, and dentistry. It had a capacity of 139 beds. In 1920, acquisition of the nearby Dental Building increased its bed capacity to 205 and provided four more operating rooms. The additional building was named the Worrall Annex.

The main Worrall was built as a nurses' home. Because of wartime demands, the Kahler Corporation instituted the Colonial Hospital Training School for Nurses in 1918. The Worrall Hospital was constructed shortly after as the nursing school's dormitory. Before it could be used, patient needs converted the building into the specialized Worrall Hospital.

The Worrall Hospital functioned as part of the Kahler Corporation's hospital group in Rochester for some years. After the Rochester Methodist Hospital Corporation purchased and used these facilities for some years, the Worrall Hospital was demolished to make way for Mayo's Guggenheim and Hilton buildings.

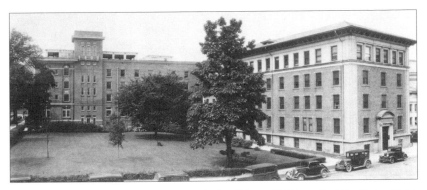

The Kahler Corporation opened the Worrall Hospital (left) in 1919 on the site of today's Hilton and Guggenheim Buildings. The nearby Dental Building was acquired by Kahler in 1920 and became the Worrall Annex (right). The buildings became part of Rochester Methodist Hospital in 1954.

Curie Hospital

During the summer of 1920, several local publications announced that the Kahler Corporation's recently opened radium hospital would be called the Curie Hospital. The building that housed the new facility was located next door to the newly constructed Kahler Hotel. Its ground floor contained the Fischer cafeteria. (Later the Rochester Diet Kitchen moved to that location.)

When it officially opened the middle of July 1920, the Curie Hospital had a 36-bed capacity. It was managed by the Kahler Corporation and was equipped for X-ray and radium treatments. Dr. Harry H. Bowing of Mayo was the medical director. Mae E. Cunningham was supervisor of the radium department and Miss Herron supervised the X-ray department.

During the early years, Dr. Bowing had a number of contacts with Madame Marie Sklodovska Curie. Initially, Dr. Charles H. Mayo had visited her in France. At that time, Madame Curie expressed interest in obtaining spent radium emanation ampoules to use in her work on polonium. Dr. Charlie encouraged others in her behalf. At Mayo, Dr. Bowing made considerable effort to assist her. Between 1923 and 1930, he personally contacted many of his colleagues in America to urge them to send the ampoules to her.

The Curie Hospital served Mayo patients until 1962. In that year, the Curie Pavilion opened in the subway level of the Damon Building to house Mayo's therapeutic radiology and clinical oncology program. The old Curie Hospital was razed in 1963 to make way for construction of the new Kahler Hotel annex.

With the opening of the Charlton Building in 1989, therapeutic radiology and clinical oncology moved into new quarters there.

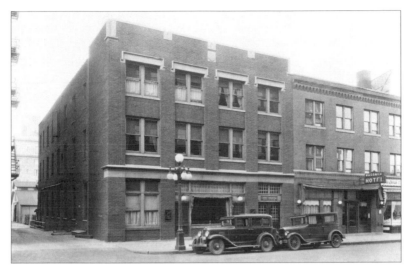

The Curie Hospital (left) was opened by the Kahler corporation in 1920. Named after Madame Curie, the hospital was equipped for X-ray and radium treatment. It was used until 1962.

Olmsted Hospital

"Where was the early Olmsted Hospital located in downtown Rochester?" is a question that surfaces in discussions about the development of Mayo's medical complex. Because of the similarity in name to today's Olmsted Community Hospital, some people assume that the first Olmsted Hospital was a forerunner of the present-day facility. The two hospitals are, however, unrelated, each having been developed by different groups at different times.

The Kahler Corporation opened the Olmsted Hospital in the spring of 1921 in the historic building that had housed the Rochester Hotel since the late 1800s. Located north of the old Lawler Theater, the three-story hotel was remodeled to provide space for the medical hospital services of Drs. L. G. Rowntree, R. Fitz, N. M. Keith, H. F. Helmholz, D. M. Berkman, G. E. Brown, S. Amberg, and R. M. Wilder. Its 65 beds provided space for a little more than a year to these sections before they moved to remodeled quarters in the old Saint Marys Hospital in July 1922. Saint Marys had opened its new surgical building that same year.

The Rochester Calorie Kitchen also opened in 1922 in the Olmsted Hospital Building. It was a forerunner of the Rochester Diet Kitchen, which provided Mayo patients with dietary instruction and meals. The kitchen remained at the Olmsted Hospital until 1926, when it moved to the Curie Hospital next to the Kahler Hotel.

The rest of the Olmsted Hospital was used as a nurses' home. In 1928, the building was moved to the northeast corner of Fifth Street and First Avenue, Southwest. It was renamed the Maxwell House and, after Rochester Methodist Hospital dropped its separate nursing program, became today's Maxwell Guest House.

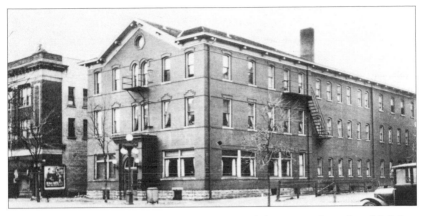

The Olmsted Hospital was opened in 1921 by the Kahler Corporation. It served as a hospital until 1922, when it became a nurses' home. The building was moved in 1928.

Subway System

When the grip of Minnesota's winter tightens, Mayo patients and personnel alike enjoy the warmth and convenience of Mayo's subway system. The present system of underground passages has evolved from the tunnel that linked Mayo's 1914 Building with the newly opened Kahler Hotel.

In the fall of 1921, the 12-story Kahler Hotel and Hospital was opened on the northeast corner of Second Avenue and First Street, Southwest. The new structure was a multipurpose facility. Its upper floors were devoted to hospital activities, and the lower levels were split between convalescent and regular hotel accommodations.

About the time the Kahler opened, a simple, white-tiled tunnel linked it and the Clinic's 1914 Building. Patients and employees moved easily between the Kahler's hospital floors and the Clinic's diagnostic facilities.

From this beginning, the Kahler Corporation extended its subway connections to the Curie Hospital and Fischer Cafeteria, the Damon Hotel, the Colonial Hospital, and the Worrall Hospital and Annex between 1921 and 1923. By 1924, work was underway on Kahler's link to the Zumbro Hotel.

When plans were developed for the Clinic's 1928 Plummer Building and its companion Franklin Heating Station, a dual-purpose tunnel was developed that accommodated both utilities and people. Since the Kahler and Mayo were joint owners of the Franklin, the new tunnel design linked both properties. Following completion of these facilities, the tunnel system remained essentially intact until Mayo began adding new buildings with subway connections in the years that followed World War II.

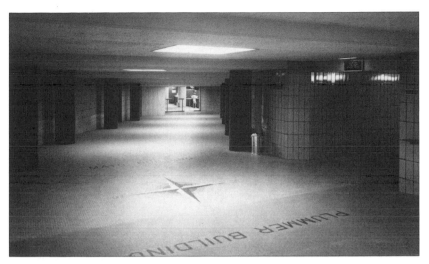

The subway system first linked Mayo's 1914 Building and the 1921 Kahler Hospital-Hotel. It has continued to expand to fit the needs of Mayo, the adjoining Kahler properties and downtown Rochester.

Rochester Methodist Hospital

Dedication ceremonies were held at the First Methodist Church and the Colonial Hospital for the newly formed Rochester Methodist Hospital on January 3, 1954. The dedicatory events took place just three days after the not-for-profit Methodist Hospital Corporation took control of the Kahler Corporation's Colonial and Worrall hospitals and related properties in the city.

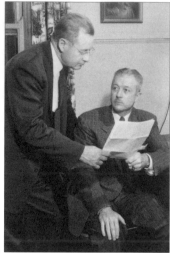

Rev. Raymond B. Spurlock (left) and Harold C. Mickey review papers for Rochester Methodist Hospital in 1954. Mickey was the first administrator of the hospital and Spurlock the first chaplain.

The event culminated efforts that began some years earlier when the Kahler Corporation decided to dispose of its hospital properties. Afterwards, such Mayo people as Drs. Arlie R. Barnes and Samuel F. Haines, as well as Harry J. Harwick, G. Slade Schuster, and Harry Blackmun (later Justice of the U.S. Supreme Court) made a variety of contacts that led to Methodist Church sponsorship of the new facility. On October 23, 1953, the first Rochester Methodist Hospital Board of Directors was formed and decided to purchase the Kahler Hospital properties.

After the acquisition and the dedication, Harold C. Mickey arrived in March 1954 to become the first administrator of the new health care facility. Rev. Raymond B. Spurlock followed him in June 1954 as the first chaplain and field representative of the hospital. In the fall, Dorothy E. Blackmun (Mrs. Harry Blackmun) helped spearhead the formation of a hospital auxiliary and became its first president in January 1955.

Construction of the modern Rochester Methodist Hospital was

begun on August 10, 1963. The completed structure was dedicated on October 21, 1966. Since then, Rochester Methodist Hospital has continued to grow and play an important role in the development of Mayo Medical Center in Rochester.

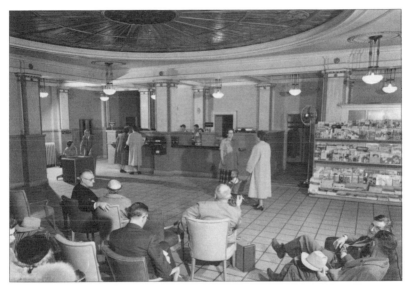

The main lobby of Rochester Methodist Hospital shortly after Methodist acquired the Kahler Hospitals in 1954.

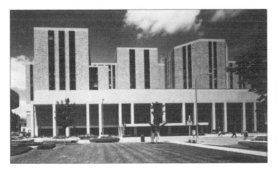

Rochester Methodist Hospital, shortly after the new building was dedicated in 1966. Construction began in 1963.

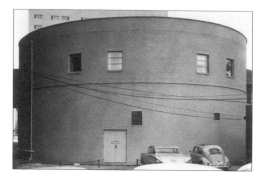

Rochester Methodist Hospital opened an experimental circular unit in 1957. The two-story facility was built with funds from the Ford Foundation and the Louis W. and Maud Hill Family Foundation. It tested the pioneering radial unit design promoted by Harold C. Mickey, hospital administrator.

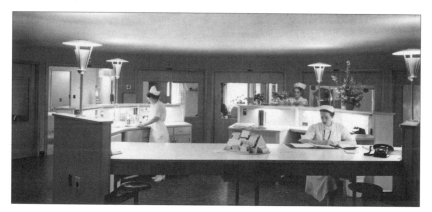

The central nursing desk in the circular or radial experimental unit at Rochester Methodist Hospital, 1957-1963. Its success led to adoption of the circular layout by other hospitals and the use of similar units in the new Rochester Methodist Hospital building in 1966.

· SECTION VI ·

Medicine and Research at Mayo

At Mayo, the ability to make astute diagnostic evaluations initially depended upon the keen clinical judgment that the elder Mayo developed through years of observation and study. With the advent of scientific medicine around the turn of the century, Dr. Mayo's sons introduced laboratory developments to make diagnosis and treatment more accurate and reliable. As clinical data accumulated from these activities, the Mayo brothers instituted research programs to collect, evaluate, and use the findings to strengthen the Clinic's ability to care for patients.

Dr. Will and Patient Care

While much of Dr. William J. Mayo's bibliography relates to surgery, it includes a number of other writings that reveal his ability to communicate. One example is an address to the graduates of the University of Minnesota Medical School on May 5, 1895. At the age of 33, Dr. Will was already making a reputation as an articulate speaker. His selection for the Minnesota commencement, instead of a prominent Eastern physician, was another step up the ladder of fame.

Despite his relative inexperience, Dr. Will did not let his audience down. Acknowledging that his "...age and limited experience do not qualify me for the task" of giving advice, he called attention to "...the kind and courteous treatment of patients which characterizes your various professors," and noted that an "interest in the welfare of those who intrust themselves to your care will bring its own reward."

Further, Dr. Will said:

I wish to call attention to the position you occupy in society, to the claim which all classes of people have upon your time and attention, and to the necessity of a broad culture upon your part to enable you to sympathize with all classes and all people in the hour of their need.

Of all the professions, the medical profession has, of necessity, always exercised a great liberality of spirit and thought toward those individuals and classes of society with whose opinions they may differ, whose actions they may condemn.

Whatever our individual beliefs may be, let us make them manifest by our acts, rather than by our words; and let us put aside all bigotry and intolerance, which would defeat the very object of our convictions by putting us out of touch with men of different views.

Let me urge you to cultivate the habit of thought and a spirit of inquiry; not to let go of the old in order to rush hurriedly after the new, but to acquire such knowledge of both the old and the new as will give you a comprehensive grasp of the whole.

Let me call your attention to the value of the experience of the older practitioner in the community in which you will work, and while you may be modern in your methods, you will soon recognize the necessity of practical knowledge.

Above all things, let me urge upon you the absolute necessity of careful examinations for the purpose of diagnosis. My own experience has been that the public will forgive you an error in treatment more readily than one in diagnosis.

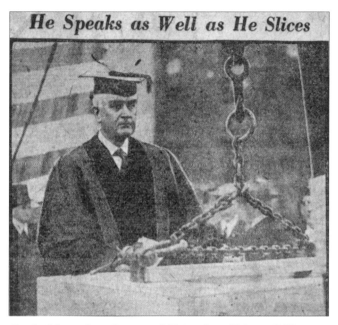

He Speaks as Well as He Slices

Both Mayo brothers exhibited striking ability on the speaker's platform — resulting from years of experience and a common-sense technique. Their presentations caught the attention of the popular news media, as well as the medical profession. This newspaper account covers Dr. Will's 1920 address to the American College of Surgeons regarding Dr. John B. Murphy, a famous surgeon of the day.

Concept of Group Medical Practice

One of the Mayo brothers' major contributions to medicine was the development of the private group practice concept. In a 1910 address, Dr. William J. Mayo detailed some of the circumstances that fostered this movement:

As we grow in learning, we more justly appreciate our dependence upon each other. The sum-total of medical knowledge is now so great and wide-spreading that it would be futile for one man to attempt to acquire, or for any one man to assume that he has, even a good working knowledge of any large part of the whole. The very necessities of the case are driving practitioners into cooperation. The best interest of the patient is the only interest to be considered, and in order that the sick may have the benefit of advancing knowledge, union of forces is necessary.

The first effort made to meet the situation was in the development of clinical specialties. Man was divided for treatment into parts, as a wagon is divided in the process of manufacture. Each part of man was assigned to those who could devote special attention to their particular portion, giving the benefit of superior skill in treatment. Unlike a wagon, man could not be treated in parts, but only as a whole, and the failure to coordinate the various specialties quickly reduced their number. It became necessary to develop medicine as a cooperative science; the clinical, the specialist, and the laboratory workers uniting for the good of the patient, each assisting in the elucidation of the problem at hand, and each dependent upon the other for support.

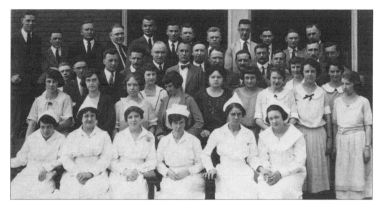

The Olmsted Hospital staff in 1922. From the first, the Mayo brothers involved all of their health-care associates in a team approach to develop the best procedures to care for the increasing number of patients.

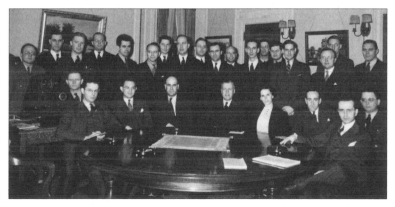

One of the regular seminars held around 1940 by Clinic physicians from different specialties. These meetings dated back to when the Mayo brothers consulted with members of the early staff in their homes. Participants reviewed the medical literature and discussed cases seen in the Clinic.

Early Mayo Surgery

Between 1889 and 1905, the Mayos were personally responsible for all operative work done at Saint Marys Hospital. Because of his senior years, Dr. William Worrall Mayo acted as consulting physician and surgeon. His two sons, Drs. William J. Mayo and Charles H. Mayo, were the attending staff and performed most of the operations.

During this pioneer period, the Mayos had a number of interns or surgical assistants who helped with the varied procedures that they undertook. The Mayos set standards for general surgery at the future Clinic during these years and also initiated work in what later became some of the Clinic's surgical specialties.

Between September 30, 1889, and January 1, 1893, the first report of Saint Marys Hospital shows that among the 1,037 patients, only 382 received medical treatment. In the years that followed, surgery continued to grow at the hospital until in 1904, when there were 3,131 operations and only 14 patients treated medically.

To handle this situation, the Mayos opened a third operating room at Saint Marys in 1905. Dr. E. Starr Judd took charge of this room. Like a number of the early surgeons, Dr. Judd was personally trained by the Mayos. He was Dr. Charlie's assistant for two years and remained his first assistant for some time later. Dr. Judd's appointment in 1905 began the development of Mayo's surgical staff.

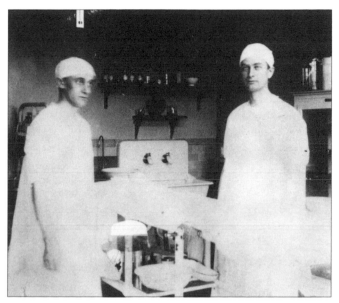

Dr. Charlie (left) and Dr. Will in the first operating room at Saint Marys Hospital.

Sister Mary Joseph

In addition to the deaths of the Mayo brothers in 1939, the Mayo staff also mourned the demise of Sister Mary Joseph Dempsey on March 29, 1939. She had been superintendent of Saint Marys Hospital for 47 years, and had supervised the development of the original pioneer facility into one handling some 600 patients. In addition, she had worked across the operating room table from Dr. William J. Mayo as his first assistant in surgery for some 25 years. According to Dr. Will, she easily ranked first among his many talented assistants.

Sister Mary Joseph, originally Julia Dempsey, was born in Salamanca, New York, on May 14, 1856. Her parents, Mr. and Mrs. Patrick Dempsey, brought the family to Olmsted County just before the Civil War. The Dempseys settled in Haverhill Township, where they raised seven children.

In 1878, Julia Dempsey entered the Sisters of the Third Order Regular of Saint Francis of the Congregation of Our Lady of Lourdes of Rochester, Minnesota. She took the name of Sister Mary Joseph and became one of three Dempsey women to join the Catholic charitable order. She advanced in the order's work and became director of the congregation's mission school in Ashland, Kentucky. After serving three years, Mother Alfred Moes, the order's founder, requested that she return to Rochester to work in their new hospital.

Sister Mary Joseph soon learned the necessary nursing skills and advanced to become superintendent of the growing hospital within a few years. In 1906, she founded Saint Marys School of Nursing. Over the years, her devotion to her church and her concern about quality patient care won her many friends among patients, no matter what their denomination.

Sister Mary Joseph's death in 1939 at the age of 82 was but a few months short of the October groundbreaking for a new medical unit at the hospital (today's Francis Building). The 1922 surgical building at Saint Marys Hospital was named the Joseph Building in her honor in 1978.

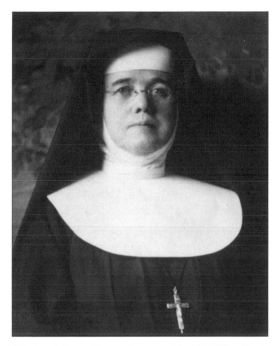

Sister Mary Joseph was Dr. Will's first assistant in surgery for some 25 years at Saint Marys Hospital. She also was the pioneer hospital administrator and founder of Saint Marys School of Nursing. She died in 1939, the same year as the Mayo brothers.

Early Clinic Visitor

Over the years, reports have appeared in various publications regarding the Mayo brothers' work in Rochester. Such accounts often record the impressions gained by a physician or patient during a Clinic visit.

In 1908, Dr. William L. Conklin reported on a Rochester stay. His remarks are interesting because of the parallels between that era and our own. The Mayo brothers were then in their mid-40s. Dr. William J. Mayo had just served as president of the American Medical Association. The brothers' practice stood on the threshold of the most ambitious expansion to date.

Within a few years, the first group practice of medicine building would be open. On Rochester's outskirts, Saint Marys Hospital was about to double its bed capacity to 300 and, in the downtown, new hospital facilities would be developed that would initially add another 240 beds. Here is Dr. Conklin's account of those exciting times:

Rochester, Minnesota, is a thriving town of about 6,000 inhabitants. It is sometimes jokingly spoken of as a 'Mayotown,' and there can be no doubt that the Mayo brothers have made the town famous.

. . . nowhere else, so far as I know, are there two surgeons who are not teachers in a medical college, yet who have the daily compliment paid them . . . of a visit from 20 to 30 doctors from all over the country. It is hard, perhaps impossible, to fully account for the remarkable growth and success . . . No doubt it is due in some degree to the fact that their father, now 80 years old, was a surgeon before them, and that they grew up in and with the great western country, with surgical cases increasing in number . . .

But the men themselves are the great cause of their success. They are strong men . . . and indefatigable workers. Added to these traits, they possess to an unusual degree the simplicity of manner . . . They talk to the doctors about them in an easy, friendly way, always ready, even anxious, to impart knowledge, but never showing egotism or assuming superiority. In watching them operate, one is impressed with their evident honesty and the conscientious and painstaking character of all their work, never operating to the gallery, but always with the patient's best good as the supreme object of attainment. Their work is practically all done at Saint Marys Hospital, . . . which is pleasantly situated just out of the town. A large addition is now being built.

The two operating rooms are on the top floor and are well lighted. In one corner of each room a sort of scaffolding or framework of gas pipe is built, onto which the 20 or 30 visiting doctors climb. The arrangement is such as to utilize the available room to the best advantage, but standing or sitting, gas pipe would become tiresome if there were not so much of interest to see. No one thinks of complaining, however, unless the man in front of him forgets and obscures his vision by standing up. The identity of the patients is absolutely unknown to those who witness the operations.

From 8 in the morning till 1 or about that, operations follow each other in quick succession. The aim is to begin the anaesthetic in one room while an operation is in progress in the other, but quite often both brothers are operating at the same time.

One of the unique features of the work at Rochester is the Surgeon's Club. All doctors who visit the clinic are expected to become members of this club. It meets every afternoon, in a pleasant room down town, and discusses for about two hours the work of the morning.

In this work of the Surgeon's Club, as in all the work of the operating room and hospital, everything is done in a very systematic way and much more is accomplished than would otherwise be possible.

On the lower floor of the building in which the Surgeon's Club meets are the offices of the Drs. Mayo, and their partner Dr. Graham, who has charge of all medical examinations and is one of the visiting physicians of Saint Marys Hospital. There is a large corps of assistants, including specialists in almost every branch of medicine. This office is open all day, and the Mayo brothers are there during all or part of the afternoon.

I am told that there is an average of 74 new patients each day. One day during my visit there were 110 patients and their friends in the waiting room or large hall which is used for that purpose, beside those who were then in the various private offices. Most of the cases which come there from out of town are surgical in character . .

During the five days I was at the hospital, there were 110 patients operated on . . . Some of these operations are done by Dr. Judd, who assists Dr. Charles Mayo, or 'Charlie' as he is often called. Dr. Judd is a very skillful operator, and when the addition to the hospital is completed, he is to have an operating room of his own.

During the five days of arduous work, I did not hear a single impatient word or see the least evidence of that which is sometimes noticed, but very undesirable in the operating room — hurry. These things I did not see, as well as those which I did see, impressed me with the greatness and goodness of the men.

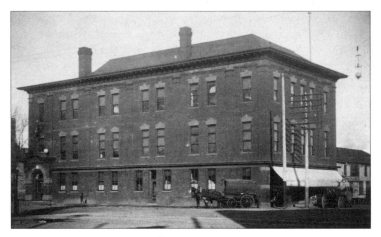

The Mayo diagnostic offices were located in the Masonic Temple in downtown Rochester. White curtains covered the windows of their first-floor offices.

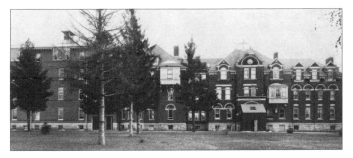

Saint Marys Hospital, about 1906. The hospital expanded west of the original building (right) in 1909 and doubled its capacity to provide 300 beds.

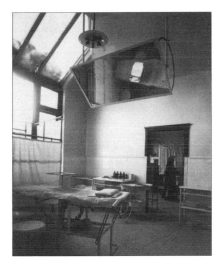

An operating room at Saint Marys Hospital around 1908. The stands for visiting physicians (left) were covered with white curtains. The overhead mirror could be positioned to allow visitors the best possible view.

Early Mayo X-Ray

In December 1895, William Conrad Roentgen, a German physicist, announced his accidental discovery of a "new kind of ray." Roentgen was fascinated with this X-ray, as he called it, especially its ability to penetrate flesh and record the details on a photographic plate.

The news of his announcement spread rapidly and, soon after, X-ray machines appeared at fairs, exhibitions, and various physicians' offices. In Rochester, Dr. J. Grosvenor Cross bought one of the new machines in February 1896. He made his first successful picture of his wife's hand after she sat for an exposure of three hours. He demonstrated the technology to the Southern Minnesota Medical Association and soon received referrals from area physicians.

The Mayo brothers were among those interested in the diagnostic possibilities of the new machine. When a little boy who had swallowed a vest buckle came for treatment, they used Dr. Cross's equipment to determine its location and how best to remove it. Dr. Cross made two pictures called skiagraphs, which showed a clear outline of the buckle and the direction of its prongs. Afterwards, Dr. Charlie successfully removed the buckle through an incision in the boy's esophagus.

Before Dr. Cross relocated in the Twin Cities, he did additional work for the Mayos. In 1900, Dr. Charlie saw a new type of X-ray machine demonstrated. Designed by the Wagner brothers of Chicago, it was said to be safer and faster than the older models. Dr. Charlie was impressed and ordered one.

Upon receiving the machine, the Mayo brothers experimented to determine what actually made it work. X-ray devices of that era had flashing lights and threw off sparks to impress patients. The Mayos would have none of these theatrics and replaced those parts with wooden pegs.

Initially, Dr. Charlie did most of the X-ray work. Like many early users, he carried scars of burns he received for the rest of his life. Dr. Christopher Graham also used the machine on occasion. Soon after the arrival of Dr. Henry S. Plummer in 1901, the X-ray machine became part of his activities as he developed Mayo's diagnostic laboratories.

In 1909, the roentgen-ray laboratory began its present-day development when Dr. Vernon J. Willey was placed in charge of the section. Rooms were made available in a new building connecting the recently erected Mayo library and the Mayo offices in the Masonic Temple. In 1911, Dr. Willey resigned because of illness, and Dr. John H. Selby was placed in charge. He left in 1913 for private practice in Washington, D.C. Dr. Alexander B. Moore, his assistant, carried on the work until the laboratory was ready to move to the south wing of the new Clinic building. Dr. Russell B. Carman was placed in charge of the Section on Roentgenology in 1913 with Dr. Moore, his associate. Before his untimely death in 1926, Dr. Carman laid the basis for today's Department of Diagnostic Radiology at Mayo. Since then, Mayo radiology has become a leader in using the latest technological developments in visualizing the organs of the body for diagnostic purposes.

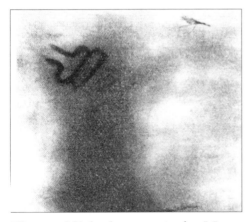

First published account of a Mayo case using x-ray to diagnose and locate a small swallowed object. *Northwestern Lancet* **17:92,1897.**

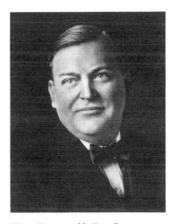

Dr. Russell B. Carman joined Mayo in 1913 as head of the Section on Roentgenology.

Laboratory Development

On January 1, 1905, Dr. Louis B. Wilson joined Mayo to organize and develop the pathologic, clinical, and experimental laboratories. Under his direction, laboratory work began in clinical pathology, gastric analysis, general pathology, surgical pathology, bacteriology, experimental surgery, biochemistry, photography, and the necropsy service.

In January 1905, laboratory space at Mayo consisted of three rooms, one of which was unequipped. The rooms were assigned to the clinical laboratory in the Masonic Temple and the gastric laboratory in Saint Marys Hospital. The staff consisted of Dr. Wilson and Helen Berkman.

Shortly after Dr. Wilson's arrival, a laboratory room near the operating rooms at Saint Marys was fitted up for pathologic and bacteriologic work. A room in the hospital's basement was designated for necropsies.

In 1908, experimental surgery was further developed by equipping six rooms in Dr. Wilson's barn. The barn was located behind his house on Fourth Street, Southwest, not far from Saint Marys.

The erection of the 1914 Mayo Clinic Building helped to centralize and provide adequate space for the growing laboratories. By 1919, patient requirements began increasing the needs for additional laboratory facilities, so that by 1925 there were 135 rooms used exclusively for laboratories, with a staff of 263, of whom 66 were physicians or other professionals.

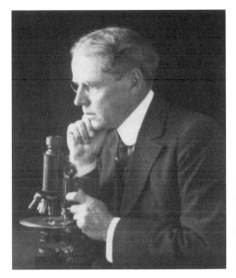

Dr. Louis B. Wilson joined Mayo in 1905. He was a leader in Mayo's laboratory development and later was the first head of Mayo's graduate school program.

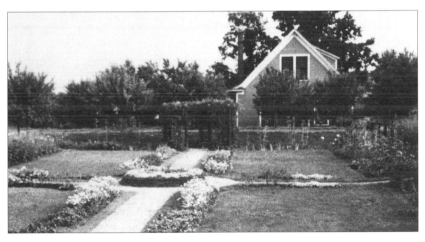

As part of Dr. Wilson's efforts to develop Mayo's research laboratories, he found that Saint Marys Hospital had little space for experimental surgery and pathology. In 1908, Dr. Wilson outfitted the upstairs area of the barn behind his home for this pioneering work. Research activity remained there until the Mayo Clinic Building opened in 1914.

Early Pediatrics at Mayo

Around the turn of the century, the specialty of pediatrics gradually became recognized, as medical schools established departmental chairs in the field and special hospitals opened to handle the needs of children. At Mayo, the care of children was a significant part of the early practice. Both Mayo brothers prepared medical papers that contained data compiled while treating the younger patient. As the Mayo practice grew, Dr. Christopher Graham became one of the early consultants who often treated children.

In 1906 Dr. Herbert Z. Giffin arrived at the Clinic, where he assisted Dr. Graham for a time. After he was named head of his own section in medicine, Dr. Giffin soon became the primary consultant in pediatrics at Mayo. When Dr. Alexander Archibald joined the Giffin section in 1911, he formed a subsection responsible for the care of children.

Dr. Archibald became head of Mayo's first Section on Pediatrics in 1916, but his tenure was interrupted by military service beginning in 1917. During that period, Dr. Rood Taylor served as head of the Section on Pediatrics. With the return of Dr. Archibald to Mayo from the military in 1919, he again became head of the section. After a year, Dr. Archibald resigned. Dr. Henry F. Helmholz was then named head of a more extensive pediatrics section in 1921. Since that time, the section has continued its growth in caring for Mayo's pediatric patients.

240

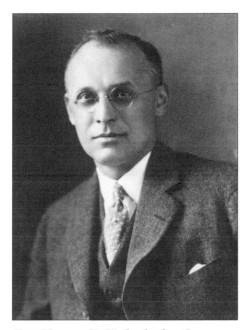

Dr. Henry F. Helmholz, Sr., was named head of a more extensive Section on Pediatrics in 1921. He founded the present-day work in pediatrics at Mayo. Before him, Drs. Alexander Archibald and Rood Taylor had been involved for short periods with pediatric care at Mayo.

Medical Records at Mayo

On July 1, 1907, Dr. Henry S. Plummer and Mabel Root inaugurated Mayo's excellent system of patient registration and medical record-keeping. The unit record was central to the new system. It brought together all the patient's medical data in a dossier filed under a number assigned during the patient's first visit. This simple system was basic to the development of Mayo's rich collection of clinical information that has supported innumerable scientific studies.

After he joined the Clinic in 1901, Dr. Plummer observed that the clinical data were scattered among the various ledgers kept by individual physicians and in the case books housed at Saint Marys Hospital. It was increasingly awkward and cumbersome to assemble data about patients and their previous Clinic visits, especially as new registrations continued their upward spiral.

After studying the situation, Dr. Plummer received approval to employ Mabel Root, a Rochester native, to assist him. Dr. Plummer trained her and, during the summer of 1907, she began creating the new record collection in six wooden files housed in the old Masonic Temple offices.

Introduction of the new system went well. As older patients returned, Mabel Root gave them the next number in her series. The data from relevant previous visits was then located and copied for insertion into the file.

Initially, Dr. Plummer envisioned batching the numbers after they reached the 100,000 mark. For this reason, early registration numbers were prefixed by the letter "A." It was tentatively planned to start over with a second series of 100,000 prefixed by the letter "B" and so on. Wisdom showed that this would cause confusion, so the series was allowed to grow in simple numerical sequence. Today, more than four million registration numbers have been used, with Mayo Clinic Jacksonville's first block of numbers beginning with 4,500,000 and Mayo Clinic Scottsdale with patient number 4,749,999. All Mayo group practice numbers are an integral part of the basic series begun in 1907.

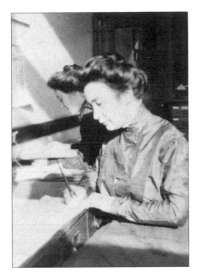

Mabel Root assisted Dr. Henry S. Plummer in establishing Mayo's system for keeping patient records in 1907. She was a Rochester native.

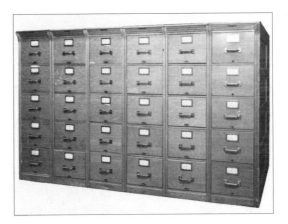

In 1907, the Plummer-Root medical record file started with these six wooden cabinets, originally kept in the Masonic Temple. Today, more than four million records fill many shelves in the Harwick Building.

General Surgery and Dr. Beckman

In 1907, Dr. Emil H. Beckman joined the growing Mayo staff as a junior surgeon. A native of Iowa, he received his M.D. degree from the University of Minnesota in 1901. After graduation, he served with the Minnesota State Board of Health laboratory (1901-1905). Dr. Beckman was chief physician of Minneapolis City Hospital and city physician of Minneapolis before coming to Mayo.

At the Clinic, Dr. Beckman first had the task of dressing the wounds of convalescent patients who were scattered in boarding houses and hotels all over Rochester. Afterward, he acted as surgical assistant, chiefly to Dr. Charles H. Mayo and occasionally to Dr. William J. Mayo. In 1911, he took charge of the new operating room number 4 at Saint Marys Hospital. He had previously shared Dr. Judd's operating room. As Mayo's fourth general surgeon, Dr. Beckman soon became known for his skill and uncanny surgical judgment. One Scottish surgeon described his work as "perfect as a professional's golf."

He played a prime role in the early development of Mayo's graduate medical school. He was chairman of the education committee charged with supervising the new program. Dr. Beckman first suggested the use of the term "fellow" for its enrollees.

In surgery, Dr. Beckman handled many operations on the brain and nervous system that others avoided. He became skilled in removing tumors of the spinal cord and was regarded as one of the gentlest and safest surgeons. He unfortunately contracted a severe infection, apparently stemming from his patient activities, and died in 1916.

Dr. Beckman's untimely death shocked the community, and more than 1,200 people attended his funeral. Out of respect, Mayo Clinic closed for several hours while his service was in progress.

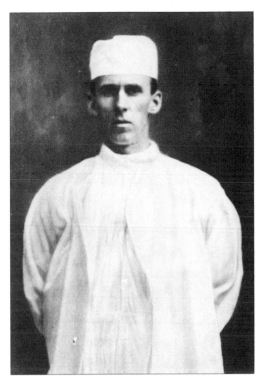

Dr. Emil H. Beckman joined Mayo as a junior surgeon in 1907. He took charge of operating room number 4 at Saint Marys Hospital in 1911. Before his death in 1916, he became known as a skilled surgeon and helped establish neurosurgery as a specialty at Mayo.

Ophthalmology

Dr. Carl Fisher became the first head of the Section on Ophthalmology at Mayo in 1909. A native of Minnesota, he received the M.D. degree from Harvard University in 1905 and served several internships in ophthalmology and otology in the Boston area.

The diagnostic work of the new section initially took place in the Mayo offices in the original Masonic Temple. With the opening of the 1914 Mayo Clinic Building, the section moved to the second floor of the new building's north wing. It remained there until rooms became available in the Zumbro Hotel Annex in 1922.

Dr. Fisher began his work in ophthalmic surgery in Room 4 of Saint Marys Hospital. Dr. Beckman, a general surgeon, regularly used the room, so Dr. Fisher had to do his surgical procedures early in the morning. Around 1912 or 1913, additional surgical and hospital space became available in the Cook Hotel in downtown Rochester, and the ophthalmology hospital service relocated there. When the Colonial Hospital became available sometime after 1915, the hospital service shifted again. Then, in 1919, the Worrall Hospital opened, and ophthalmology moved to the new facility, where it remained for several decades.

Dr. Fisher remained head of the section until he left for service in the U.S. Army in 1917. Dr. William L. Benedict was appointed the new head of the section in May 1917. During this pioneering period, Dr. John J. W. Looney succeeded Dr. Granger in the section in 1914. With the inauguration of the Mayo Graduate School program, he became the first fellow in ophthalmology. He left the Clinic in 1918.

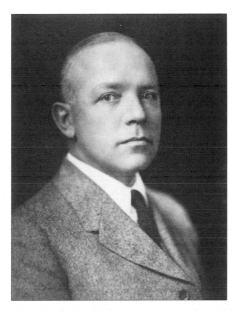

Dr. Carl D. Fisher was appointed
first head of the Section on
Ophthalmology in 1909. He
initiated ophthalmic surgery in
room 4 at Saint Marys Hospital,
where he worked around the
surgical schedule of Dr. E. H.
Beckman.

Ophthalmology and Dr. Granger

The early work in ophthalmology at the Clinic initially centered on activities of Dr. Charles Horace Mayo, the younger of the Mayo brothers. By 1895, Dr. Charlie was handling most operations on the eye, ear, nose, throat, bones, and joints. Along with these surgical activities, he did eye refractions and took care of ophthalmologic diseases. In 1898, Dr. Gertrude Booker became Dr. Charlie's clinical assistant in treating diseases of the eye, ear, nose, and throat. She later took charge of eye refractions at Mayo.

Dr. Booker was a native of Quincy, Minnesota. She received her M.D. degree from the University of Minnesota in 1897. Before joining Mayo, she was in private practice in Dover and Eyota.

In 1900, Dr. Booker married George W. Granger. He was a prominent Rochester attorney and an original incorporator of Mayo Properties Association, today's Mayo Foundation.

Dr. G. Booker Granger remained active in Mayo's eye refraction work until 1914. She resigned that year to become health officer of Rochester under Dr. Charlie's direction. Dr. Booker Granger continued as health officer for two years. She then opened a limited private practice in refractions of the eye. She died in Rochester in 1928.

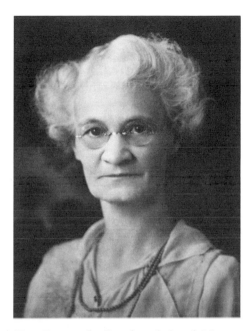

Dr. Gertrude Booker joined Mayo in 1898 to assist Dr. Charlie with his eyework. She later took charge of eye refractions. After her marriage to Judge Granger, she remained at Mayo until 1914.

Electrocardiography

The use of electrocardiograms in the study of heart conditions began at Mayo by Dr. John M. Blackford under Dr. Henry S. Plummer's supervision. Dr. Blackford entered the Clinic in 1911 as an assistant in pathology. After inaugurating the electrocardiographic service, Dr. Blackford trained Dr. Frederick A. Willius, a new Clinic fellow, to assist him in 1915. Dr. Willius took over the laboratory in 1917, when Dr. Blackford left for Seattle. In 1922, Dr. Willius established a section on medicine with a special interest in cardiology.

Mayo's first electrocardiograph unit was ordered from England in 1912. The Cambridge device did not arrive until 1914 because it was custom-made and required considerable assembly time. Early users of the instrument remembered that it was large, slow to use, and had a complicated optical assembly that was subject to alignment problems.

The Cambridge electrocardiograph was the fundamental equipment in the new laboratory, located in two adjoining rooms in the north corridor of what later became the third floor of the 1914 Building. It was installed in a darkroom. The connecting leads from the instrument passed through the wall into the next room where the patient waited. Electrodes were attached to the patient's limbs, which rested in shallow metal pans filled with a concentrated saline solution. The metal pans often suffered corrosion problems. After the reading was taken, the glass photographic plate on which it had been recorded went to the Section on Photography for processing and then returned to the Electrocardiographic Laboratory for interpretation.

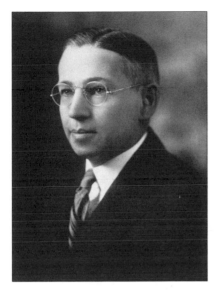

Dr. Frederick A. Willius established a section on medicine with a special interest in cardiology in 1922. He had been placed in charge of Mayo's electrocardiographic service in 1917.

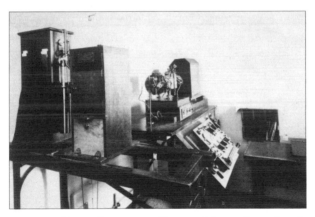

Mayo's first electrocardiographic unit arrived from England in 1914. The Cambridge equipment was slow and awkward to use.

Clinical Pathology

In the spring of 1911, Dr. Arthur H. Sanford of Marquette University was considering entering the United States Public Health Service when a letter from Mayo informed him of a newly created laboratory post. The young teacher of physiology accepted the opportunity and became Mayo's bacteriologist, effective June 1, 1911.

Arriving at Mayo, Dr. Sanford opened his clinical pathology laboratory in the small building adjoining the first Masonic Temple. The laboratory quickly outgrew the space, so enlarged quarters were designed for the 1914 Clinic Building.

As director of clinical laboratories, Dr. Sanford helped develop Mayo's excellence in this activity. He was the head of the Section on Clinical Pathology until 1946.

During his career at Mayo, Dr. Sanford became widely known and honored in his field. One of his major contributions was the coauthorship with Dr. James C. Todd of *Clinical Diagnosis by Laboratory Methods*. The work went through many editions and became a classic publication. Dr. Sanford collaborated with Dr. Charles Sheard of Mayo in development of the Sheard and Sanford Photoelometer, a pioneering instrument for the quantitative determination of blood constituents.

Dr. Sanford was active in a variety of Clinic and community activities. He retired from Mayo in 1949 and died in Rochester in 1959.

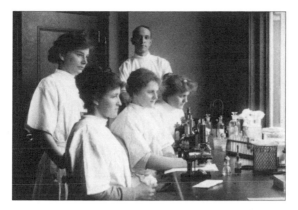

Dr. Arthur H. Sanford, standing rear, came to Mayo in 1911 to set up the clinical pathology laboratory. The technicians pictured with Sanford around 1920, are, from left: Hazel Ungemack, Lola Callahan, Madge Sinclair, and Elizabeth Cronin.

Neurology

Dr. Walter D. Shelden arrived in Rochester to head Mayo's first Section on Neurology in August 1913. At the time, Dr. Shelden was a mature physician who was 43 years old. He received his M.D. degree from Rush Medical College in 1895. After entering private practice in Wisconsin, he spent two years studying in Vienna. Upon his return to Minnesota in 1903, he again entered private practice while holding a number of academic appointments beginning in 1906. He was a clinical professor at the University of Minnesota Medical School when he joined Mayo.

While at the university, Dr. Shelden acquired a reputation as a diagnostician and a clinical teacher with a particular interest in neurology. At Mayo, he emphasized the importance of a general physical examination as a requisite for the neurologic patient. Dr. Shelden also favored the close collaboration between ophthalmology and neurology, feeling that an eye examination was beneficial. As a result of his medical emphasis, Dr. Shelden helped foster the development of a neurology section that became strong in the neurological sciences and offered educational opportunities. In July 1915, Dr. Charles H. Doe became the first fellow to spend time in the section. Since then, medical students have regularly rotated through neurology.

About 1918, Dr. Shelden developed a half-sheet form on which to record findings of the neurologic examination. Dr. H. W. Woltman expanded the form to a full neurologic sheet around 1922. Over the years, Mayo's neurologic record sheet has continued to evolve and, with modifications, has been useful to practitioners outside the Clinic.

Dr. Shelden, or "Pop" as he became affectionately known, had many interests and skills besides medicine. In his collegiate days, he played on Wisconsin's first football team and on its baseball team. He enjoyed working with wood and was a proficient wood-carver. In Rochester, he became known for his love of golfing. He helped develop the Rochester Golf and Country Club and personally planted hundreds of trees on the club's grounds. A stone monument in memory of his service was placed near the club's first tee in 1949.

Before stepping down as neurology head in 1930, Dr. Shelden was associated with the following pioneer consultants in the section: Drs. Henry W. Woltman (1919-1956); Frederick P. Moersch (1921-1956); Harry L. Parker (1925-1934, 1945-1959); John P. Doyle (1921-1931); and Lloyd H. Ziegler (1926-1930). Dr. Shelden remained a senior consultant in the section until his retirement in 1943. He died in 1946.

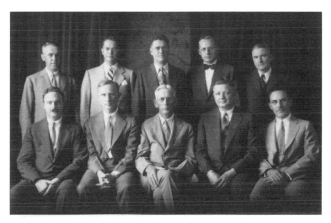

Dr. Shelden in 1931, with members of the Section on Neurology and their associates in surgery, ophthalmology, and pathology. Back row, from left: Drs. James W. Kernohan (pathologist), Winchell McK. Craig (neurosurgeon), John B. Doyle (neurologist), Walter I. Lillie (ophthalmologist), James R. Learmonth (neurosurgeon). Front row, from left: Drs. Harry Lee Parker (neurologist), Henry W. Woltman (neurologist), Walter D. Shelden (neurology section head), Alfred W. Adson (neurosurgeon), and Frederick P. Moersch (neurologist).

Thoracic Surgery

Dr. Samuel Robinson arrived at Mayo in January 1915 to develop the Section on Thoracic Surgery. Besides heading the new section, he was also first assistant in general surgery. Before coming to Mayo, Dr. Robinson received an M.D. degree from Harvard (1902) and interned at Massachusetts General Hospital, Boston (1903). He was in private practice from 1903 to 1912 and worked in a tuberculosis sanitarium from 1912 to 1915. Dr. Robinson published some 20 papers related to thoracic surgery before coming to Mayo.

Dr. Robinson's tenure at the Clinic was short-lived. With the advent of World War I, he entered the U.S. Army in 1917 and served as chief of surgical service at Letterman General Hospital, Presidio, California. After military service, he remained in private surgical practice in California.

While Dr. Robinson was in the service, thoracic operations at Mayo took place in various sections of general surgery. On January 1, 1919, Dr. Carl A. Hedblom became head of the Section on General and Thoracic Surgery. Dr. Ambrose L. Lockwood followed him in 1921. Dr. Lockwood left Mayo in 1922 to establish the Lockwood Clinic in Toronto, Canada, and Dr. Hedblom again assumed leadership of the section. He remained at the Clinic until 1924, when he left to become Professor of Surgery at the University of Wisconsin. Dr. Stuart W. Harrington then took over the section. He had been head of a section of general surgery at Mayo since 1920.

Dr. Harrington entered the Clinic in 1914 and became a fellow in surgery. In 1920, he received the M.S. degree in surgery from Mayo's graduate program in medicine. During his training, he spent considerable time as a surgical assistant to Drs. Charles H. Mayo and E. Starr Judd.

Because of the limited time each of his predecessors spent as section head, Dr. Harrington might properly be thought of as the founder of thoracic surgery at Mayo. During his 30 years as section head, he became noted for his surgical skills and productivity. He enjoyed long hours in the operating rooms and often would work until midnight.

As a young man, he achieved fame in football as an All-American halfback known as "Tack" at the University of Pennsylvania. His father did not approve of his choice of medicine as a career, and Dr. Harrington worked as a counselor in youth camps and as a coach to earn tuition money for medical school.

Following Dr. Harrington's retirement in 1954, he and his wife, Gertrude Jones, remained staunch supporters of Mayo's programs. Childless, they left a significant legacy to Mayo after their passing. The Stuart W. Harrington Professor of Surgery in Mayo Foundation is one example of their benefaction.

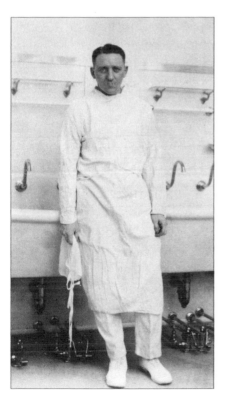

Dr. Stuart W. (Tack) Harrington was head of the Section on General and Thoracic Surgery from 1924 until 1954. A series of surgeons had previously held short-term appointments in the specialty, dating back to 1915. Dr. Harrington might be considered the founder of thoracic surgery at Mayo.

Thoracic Diseases Diagnostic Section

On June 1, 1918, Dr. Willis S. Lemon was appointed the first head of a new section of medicine. The section had a special emphasis in thoracic diseases. Dr. Lemon had arrived at the Clinic the year before to serve as an assistant in medicine.

Born in Canada, Dr. Lemon received his M.B. degree from the University of Toronto in 1905. After an internship and a research appointment in Toronto, he served as an intern in the Canadian National Sanatorium for Tuberculosis. Coming to the United States in 1909, he practiced privately in Illinois before he joined Mayo in 1917.

The new diagnostic section that Dr. Lemon formed in 1918 complemented the work of the new Section on General and Thoracic Surgery organized by Dr. Samuel Robinson in 1915. Activity in this surgical section had doubled in the three years between its formation and the establishment of its supporting diagnostic section.

In 1923, Dr. Porter P. Vinson joined Dr. Lemon in the thoracic diseases section. He came to the Clinic in 1916 and worked with both of the Plummer brothers in their diagnostic activities. Dr. Vinson assisted Dr. Henry S. Plummer in bronchoscopy and esophagoscopy, and he took complete charge of this work in the Lemon section.

Besides Drs. Lemon and Vinson, the early consultants in the thoracic diseases section were: Drs. Fred W. Gaarde (1920), Herman J. Moersch (1926), Harry G. Wood (1926), H. Corwin Hinshaw (1936), and Herbert W. Schmidt (1938).

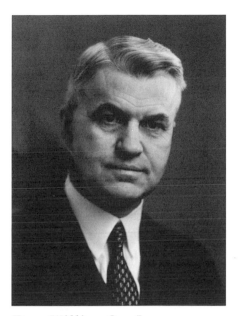

Dr. Willis S. Lemon was appointed first head of a new section on medicine with a special interest in thoracic diseases in 1918. The new section worked closely with Mayo's thoracic surgeons.

Dermatology

Dr. John H. Stokes organized the Section on Dermatology and Syphilology at Mayo in August 1916. A year later, Drs. Paul A. O'Leary and William H. Goeckerman joined him as first assistants.

After Dr. Stokes resigned in 1924, Dr. Paul A. O'Leary was appointed section head and served in that capacity until 1953. Dr. Louis A. Brunsting headed the section from 1953 to 1962 and was followed by Drs. Robert R. Kierland (1962-1970); Richard K. Winkelmann (1970-1975); Harold O. Perry (1975-1982); and the current department chairman, Sigfrid A. Muller. Syphilology was dropped from the section's name after 1958, and in 1970 the section was renamed Department of Dermatology.

Diagnostic work was first done in the east annex between the 1914 Building and the old Masonic Temple. In August 1918, dermatology moved to the seventh floor of the Zumbro Hotel Annex, where it remained until the 1928 Building was finished and North 7 became available. When the Mayo Building was completed, the section moved to its present location on the fifth floor.

Hospital service for dermatology patients was first available in the Colonial Hospital. Beginning in 1919, it relocated to the Worrall, and a year later it settled in the Worrall Annex, where it remained until Rochester Methodist Hospital was completed in 1966.

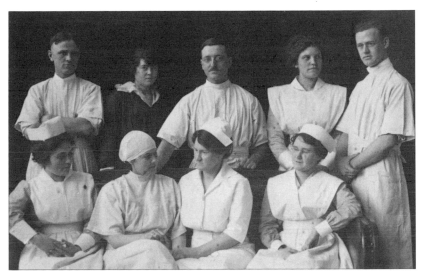

Dr. John H. Stokes, standing center, formed the Section on Dermatology and Syphilology in 1916. Those pictured around 1917 are, standing at left: Dr. James M. Hayes, unidentified, Dr. Stokes, unidentified, and Dr. Paul A. O'Leary. The individuals who are seated are unidentified.

Proctology

On February 1, 1917, Dr. Louis A. Buie entered the Mayo Graduate School as a fellow in surgery. Before his arrival, he had conducted orthopedic clinics at the University of Maryland for two years. At the conclusion of his Mayo fellowship in 1919, Dr. Buie joined Dr. Logan's section in the Clinic's Division of Medicine. He began centralizing Mayo's proctoscopic work, which had previously been done in the Section on Urology.

On April 1, 1924, Dr. Buie became the first head of Mayo's Section on Proctology. Until his retirement in 1955, he played a leading role in developing proctology as a specialty in America. Among his publications are three proctologic texts, of which he was sole author or coauthor. His 1937 book, *Practical Proctology*, was widely used in America and abroad. Dr. Buie also served as first editor of the journal *Diseases of the Colon & Rectum* from 1957 to 1967.

He developed several instruments or types of apparatus; among them were the Buie sigmoidoscope, the Buie proctoscopic table, and the Buie forceps for taking specimens of tissue for biopsy.

He was one of the founders of the American Board of Proctology and served as its president from 1934 to 1935. He was also president of the American Proctologic Society from 1927 to 1928 and again from 1934 to 1935.

Dr. Buie served as secretary treasurer of the Advisory Board for Medical Specialties from 1958 to 1970. In the American Medical Association, he was prominent between 1945 and 1961 in its Judicial Council, where he played a major role in the revision of the AMA Code of Medical Ethics.

Dr. Buie died on July 2, 1975. His son, Dr. Louis A. Buie, Jr., is a Mayo alumnus.

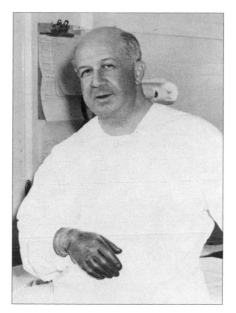

Dr. Louis A. Buie arrived at Mayo in 1917. He became the first head of the Section on Proctology in 1924.

Dental Surgery

On October 1, 1918, Boyd S. Gardner, D.D.S., arrived at Mayo to establish the Section on Dental Surgery. This unique association of dentistry and medicine began because of Dr. Charles H. Mayo's interest in dentistry and focal infection.

Before the section was formed, dental surgery had been handled in the general surgery sections and the Section on Otolaryngology and Rhinology. Dr. Gordon B. New was especially interested in the field. One dental chair was available, which Dr. A. B. Moore used for limited dental X-ray work in the Section on Roentgenology.

With Dr. Gardner's arrival, these scattered dental activities were centralized in two small rooms in a single-story building located southeast of the 1914 Clinic Building. At that time, the structure also housed other medical offices of the expanding Mayo practice. In more recent years, it served as as a garage for Clinic ambulances.

The section quickly grew. In 1921, it moved to new quarters on the ground floor of the building adjoining the Masonic Temple in downtown Rochester. A total of seven offices, two waiting rooms, and two new X-ray machines provided a more functional arrangement for the expanding activity.

With the opening of the 1928 Clinic Building, the dental section relocated to Desk S-4 in 1929. It remained there until the Mayo Building was ready for occupancy in the 1950s, and the section shifted to its present location on W-4 in the new building.

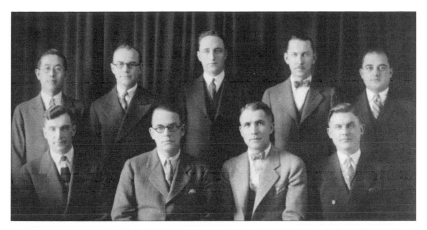

Dr. Boyd S. Gardner, seated second from left, formed the Section on Dental Surgery on October 1, 1918. Photographed with him around 1926 are, seated from left: Drs. Frank J. Vermeulin, Louie T. Austin, and Murvale Page Kendrick; standing from left: Drs. Kenji Hiyama, Burr M. McWilliams, Daniel F. Lynch, Edward C. Stafne, and James W. Thayer.

Physiotherapy

The Section on Physiotherapy was organized in November 1918 by Antoinette White, a graduate of the Sargent School for Physical Education. The new section was under the supervision of Dr. Melvin S. Henderson, head of the Section on Orthopaedic Surgery.

Initially, Antoinette White used three rooms on the second floor of the old medical library building, which stood on the northeast corner of the present Plummer Building lot. One of the upstairs rooms was an enclosed sun porch over the library entrance. An additional room on the main floor served wheelchair patients. In 1924, the section moved to the Colonial Hospital and used four rooms and a sun porch.

Rosalie Donaldson took over in 1920, and was succeeded by Mildred Elson in 1923. A branch of the section was organized in 1923 at Saint Marys Hospital. By 1926, Physiotherapy was treating more than 1,000 patients a month at Mayo.

As the section's work increased, it became too broad for Dr. Henderson to supervise, and for a time, Dr. Arthur U. Desjardins, head of the Section on Therapeutic Radiology, was responsible for physiotherapy. When Dr. Desjardins found his own specialty too demanding, he recommended Dr. Frank H. Krusen to replace him. Dr. Krusen arrived at Mayo in 1935 to set up the Section on Physical Medicine and refine the program of physical therapy.

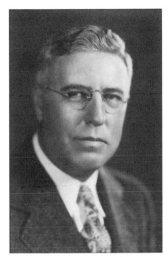

Dr. Melvin S. Henderson founded the Section on Orthopaedics at Mayo. He also began the work of physiotherapy at the Clinic in 1918.

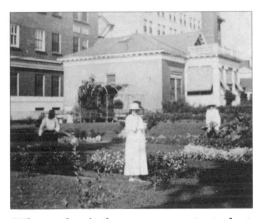

When physiotherapy was started at the Clinic in 1918, it was located on the second floor of Mayo's library building. The porch was enclosed for use by the section.

Parasitology

Dr. Thomas B. Magath came to Mayo as first assistant in clinical pathology in October 1919. At the time, he had received an invitation to join the laboratory of the Rockefeller Foundation but opted for the Mayo appointment instead. In 1921, Dr. Magath was appointed head of Mayo's Section on Parasitology and in 1946 became chairman of the Section on Clinical Pathology and the Section on Clinical Biochemistry. He became senior consultant in 1958, retired from Mayo in 1960, and died in 1981.

During his four decades of service at the Clinic, Dr. Magath became internationally known for his studies on the fish tapeworm, amebic dysentery, and hydatid disease. In Rochester, he succeeded Dr. Charles H. Mayo as city health officer from 1936 to 1941. Magath was founding editor of the *American Journal of Clinical Pathology* from 1930 to 1936. He served as president of the American Society of Clinical Pathologists in 1938, and the Minnesota Academy of Science, 1933 to 1934. During World War II, he served in the U.S. Navy and rose to the rank of commodore in 1945. He later became rear admiral in the U.S. Naval Reserve. At Mayo, he was a member of the Board of Governors from 1948 to 1956.

For three years, Dr. Magath was a close associate of Dr. Henry S. Plummer during the planning and construction of the 1928 Clinic Building. Dr. Magath became a sounding board and a developer of Dr. Plummer's ideas for the new building's internal systems for handling patients. Dr. Magath helped devise the patient's master history sheet and helped reduce the number of patient forms that had proliferated. Since he had worked his way through medical school as a printer's assistant, Dr. Magath set the type for new forms when the printer was unable to understand Dr. Plummer's instructions.

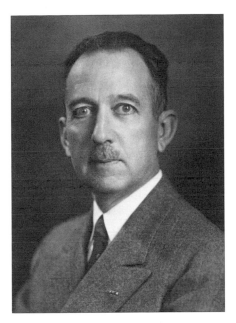

Dr. Thomas B. Magath came to
Mayo in 1919. He was appointed
head of the Section on
Parasitology in 1921.

Pathologic Anatomy

Dr. Harold E. Robertson was a major figure in the early development of the Mayo Section on Pathologic Anatomy. He was appointed head of the section on July 1, 1921. Before coming to Mayo, he was Director of the Department of Pathology, Bacteriology, and Public Health at the University of Minnesota. Dr. Robertson brought a strong conviction of the educational value of postmortem examinations to his position at Mayo. He conducted staff pathologic conferences to improve Mayo's diagnostic and treatment skills.

In addition to his regular work, Dr. Robertson authored some 150 scientific writings. He had a particular interest in tetanus and poliomyelitis. In 1925, he served as president of the American Association of Pathology and Bacteriology.

When he came to Mayo in 1921, Dr. Robertson brought Louis Richard Lundquist to head the tissue preparation laboratory. Lundquist started collecting material for a display museum. Among the first exhibits was a display of foreign bodies removed from the bronchi and esophagus by Drs. Plummer and Vinson. Later, E. L. Judah of McGill University assisted Lundquist in setting up the specimens. Some of Lundquist's pathological exhibits were displayed at national meetings. Over the years, Richard Lundquist and Dr. Robertson coauthored a series of papers on the mounting and preservation of museum specimens. These writings appeared in many scientific journals.

In 1943, Dr. Robertson became senior consultant. He died on March 8, 1946.

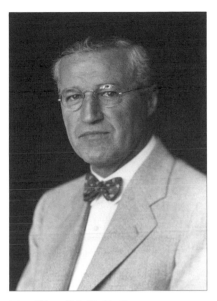

Dr. Harold E. Robertson came to Mayo in 1921. He was appointed head of the Section on Pathologic Anatomy. Dr. Robertson instituted staff pathologic conferences to help improve Mayo's diagnostic skills.

Biophysics

In 1919, Professor William Duane of Harvard University installed a small laboratory of radiophysics on the ground floor of the 1914 Clinic Building and the eighth floor of the Zumbro Annex. The new unit was primarily used for the preparation of radium in the treatment of patients.

After Professor Duane returned to Harvard, Howard C. Stearns took over the new laboratory as physicist in charge. With the completion of the Curie Hospital in 1921, the endeavor moved there. Stearns left Mayo in 1923, and Roy Kegerreis took over the laboratory post for a year.

On March 1, 1924, Dr. Charles Sheard arrived at Mayo and established the Section on Biophysics. Dr. Sheard earned the Ph.D. at Princeton University in 1912. His responsibilities included the radiophysics laboratory. With establishment of the new section, it became the first biophysics unit in a medical institution. Later in 1924, Dr. Sheard was joined by Drs. Edward J. Baldes and John M. Ort as assistants.

Between 1929 and 1933, Dr. Sheard collaborated with Dr. Arthur H. Sanford and Mr. Dana Rogers of Mayo in developing the Sheard and Sanford Photoelometer colorimeter for the quantitative determination of hemoglobin and other blood constituents. Dr. Sheard also devised an artificial larynx or voice box in 1931, which was used at Mayo for several decades.

Until his retirement in 1949, Dr. Sheard and his department consultants, fellows, and technicians developed the Mayo biophysics activity into one of America's unique enterprises.

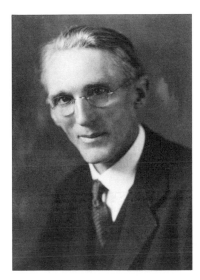

Dr. Charles Sheard established
the Section on Biophysics at Mayo
in 1924. The section was the first
of its kind in a medical
institution.

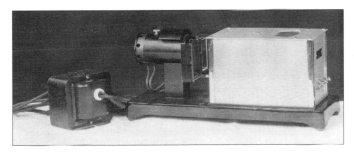

Dr. Sheard collaborated with Dr. Arthur H. Sanford
and Dana Rogers of Mayo in designing the Sheard
and Sanford Photoelometer between 1929 and 1933.
It was the first successful instrument to determine
the quantitative constituents of blood, and was
widely used in hospitals and medical laboratories.

Nurse Anesthetists

From the beginning at Saint Marys Hospital, the Mayos employed specially trained anesthetists to enhance their surgical efforts. In other hospitals of that era, rotating interns gave anesthesia with varied effectiveness.

The Graham sisters, Dinah and Edith, are the first examples of such allied health workers at Mayo, if not in America. Dinah Graham, the older sister, was a trained nurse who for a short period gave anesthetics at the hospital under Dr. A. W. Stinchfield's direction. Soon after, Edith Graham took over the administration of anesthetics along with teaching the Sisters the rudiments of nursing. Edith was also a nurse and remained as anesthetist for the Mayos until her marriage to Dr. Charlie in 1893.

Alice Magaw, graduate of a Chicago nursing school, succeeded her and continued as the only anesthetist until 1900. Over the years that followed, a series of anesthetists joined the growing numbers of Mayo surgeons. Alice Magaw, later Kessel, remained a prominent member of this pioneering group until after the Section on Anesthesia was started by Dr. John S. Lundy in 1924.

During this early period, Alice Magaw became noted for her contributions to the methodology of anesthesia. Because of the rapid expansion of surgical activities nationwide, methods of giving safe anesthetics were of great interest. The Mayo brothers had early adopted the open drop method of giving ether. Alice Magaw became an exponent of this technique and prepared several papers in which she reported highly successful results. In 1904, she addressed the state medical society on her experiences from 11,000 cases. She reported on 14,000 surgical anesthesias before the Missouri Medical Society in 1906. In her presentations, she demonstrated that anesthetics could be given with a sensitivity to the emotional and physical needs of the patient. She further reinforced the "team approach" in group practice that the Mayo brothers were so prominent in promoting.

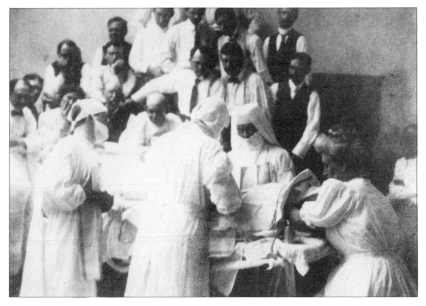

Alice Magaw giving anesthetics during surgery for Dr. Will (left) and Sister Mary Joseph at Saint Marys Hospital.

· SECTION VII ·
Education at Mayo

After their graduation from medical school in
the 1880s, the Mayo brothers kept abreast of the
latest developments by studying the literature
and visiting other medical centers. Through
these activities, the brothers continued to refine
their medical and surgical skills. As their
abilities and reputations grew, great numbers of
physicians flocked to Rochester to learn about
the brothers' methods. The demand for such
advanced training led the Mayo brothers to
found the country's first graduate program in
clinical medicine in 1915. Mayo has since
developed into a multifaceted educational center
in medicine and science.

Continuing Medical Education

Continuing medical education at Mayo has its roots in the early educational activities of the founders, Drs. William J. Mayo and Charles H. Mayo. Each of the brothers, following graduation from medical school, enrolled in postgraduate courses in New York City.

Dr. Will received his second M.D. from the New York Polyclinic for Practitioners in 1885 where he learned from one of America's leaders in antiseptic and aseptic surgery, Dr. Arpad G. Gerster. Dr. Charlie followed his brother to New York City and received his second M.D. degree from the Polyclinic in 1889.

The age of scientific medicine was unfolding and the Mayos, like many other physicians, sought a better understanding of the new insights. Advanced teaching clinics were springing up in major American cities. These activities usually featured some gifted physician or surgeon who accepted visitors for limited periods. The Mayos discovered that the quality of these programs varied greatly.

Consequently, the brothers soon established a systematic pattern of traveling to the sources of new medical knowledge. In the spring Dr. Charlie would take a trip either in America or abroad to visit some physician or medical center that held promise of new information. Following his return, Dr. Will journeyed in the fall to another location. The Mayo brothers followed this pattern for most of their careers, and frequently acknowledged the stimulus that these activities brought to the medical practice in Rochester.

During their professional travels, the Mayos discovered that some colleagues were reluctant to share their full knowledge. As a result, the brothers vowed to make their experiences readily available in Rochester without restraint. By the turn of the century, the Mayos' surgical talents and their "open-door" policy were attracting such numbers of physicians and surgeons to Rochester that visitors formed an organization in 1906 to facilitate their time in Rochester.

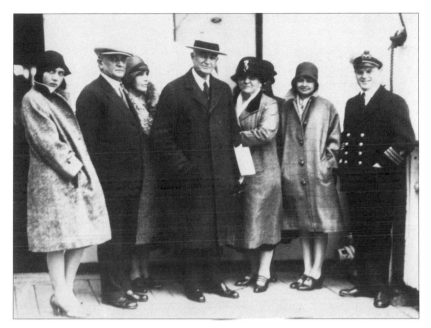

Normally, the Mayo brothers alternated between staying in Rochester and traveling to learn from other physicians in the United States or abroad. This 1929 photograph records one of the few occasions when the brothers traveled together. Dr. Charlie (left) and Dr. Will (center) stand with their wives beside them. Two of the brothers' nieces are on either side, along with the ship's officer.

The Surgeons Club

On June 7, 1906, the International Surgeons Club was organized in Rochester, Minnesota, by six surgeons who were visiting the Mayo brothers and their operating rooms at Saint Marys Hospital. The club enhanced the visits of growing numbers of surgeons who came to observe the brothers' surgical skills.

From the beginning, the Mayos maintained an "open-door" policy to other members of the medical profession. During operations, the brothers always discussed their procedures for the benefit of visitors. As the numbers of visiting surgeons grew, the Mayos introduced several improvements in their operating rooms. Movable, elevated metal stands were positioned to allow a better view of operations from the sidelines. Over the operating tables, large adjustable mirrors provided a complete view of the operating field.

The International Surgeons Club was one step that helped develop the Mayo practice into a center of learning. Dr. J. L. Wiggins of East St. Louis, Illinois, was elected first president of the temporary organization. Each Monday, new officers were elected from among those visiting. Reporters covered the surgical schedules in each operating room.

At the conclusion of the day, members of the club gathered in rented rooms in downtown Rochester to review what they had observed. Discussions were open and frank. The Mayo brothers attended only when they were asked to speak; otherwise, they did not want to influence the group's activities by being present. From time to time, other members of the Mayo staff would, on request, present lectures on topics in their fields.

Soon after the club was organized, its name was shortened to the Surgeons Club. As the numbers grew to 40 or more a day, rules of conduct were instituted for the operating rooms. The daily reporters enforced these rules for everyone's benefit. During the Club's first summer, its membership expanded to more than 300, including surgeons from throughout the United States, Canada, and several other countries.

The registration fee was $0.50; later it became $1, and then it increased to $2. These funds paid the rent for the club's meeting room adjoining Mayo offices in downtown Rochester. In time, the group rented the entire second floor of the building, and tables, chairs, and a blackboard were included among the furnishings. A local physician, Dr. J. E. Crewe, became permanent secretary of the group. He secured free copies of some medical books and periodicals for use in the rooms.

The quality of educational experiences in Rochester soon became known in the medical journals of that day. One Canadian physician, writing in the *Canada Lancet*, noted: "The little western town [is] slowly becoming the greatest postgraduate centre of the century, with possibilities unlimited." In 1919, the club changed its name to the Physicians and Surgeons Club. Its program of lectures enlarged to cover all specialties.

With the founding of Mayo Graduate School of Medicine in 1915, the club gradually became diffused as the lectures and seminars of the graduate school became opened to visitors. In time, the formalities of the club ceased, even though outside physicians continued to be welcome at Mayo.

Today, the same "open-door" attitude prevails, and those interested in advanced medical education pursue various specialty programs at Mayo Graduate School of Medicine.

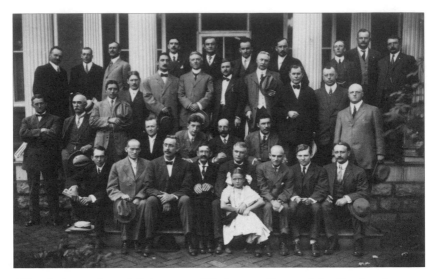

The International Surgeons Club was formed in Rochester on June 7, 1906, by visiting physicians. Later called the Surgeons Club, the informal group gathered each day to discuss the Mayos' surgical clinics at Saint Marys Hospital. This picture was taken on September 4, 1909, with Dr. Will and his youngest daughter, Phoebe, seated in the front row. The physicians with them represent 19 states, Canada, Ireland, and Scotland.

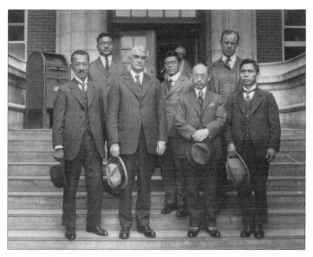

Dr. Will, second from front left, with a group of Japanese physicians at the Clinic in 1923. Many international groups visited the Clinic for varying lengths of time to observe and learn.

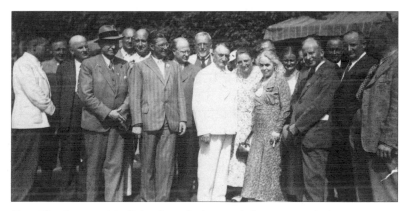

Dr. Charles and Edith, fourth from right, entertaining a group of German physicians at Mayowood, their country home. In the early years, Rochester had few large hotels, and the Mayo brothers built homes to help accommodate and entertain the many physicians who were coming to visit their surgical clinics.

Graduate Medical Education at Mayo

In February 1915, the Mayo brothers executed a series of legal agreements that founded and endowed the work of today's Mayo Graduate School of Medicine. Some years before, the brothers began searching for ways to coordinate and develop the educational activities that had emerged as part of their efforts to improve patient care at the Clinic. With encouragement from President George E. Vincent and others at the University of Minnesota, a graduate education program in clinical medicine was established in affiliation with the graduate school of the University of Minnesota.

The Mayo brothers initially endowed the undertaking with $1.5 million, the bulk of their life savings. The University of Minnesota issued a preliminary announcement of the new graduate program in September 1915, and by August 1916 the university bulletin listed 71 graduate students enrolled for the 1915-1916 school year in Mayo's advanced medicine program. On June 14, 1917, the first graduate degrees in the new curriculum were conferred on two women and two men. In 1983, Mayo Foundation became an independent degree-granting institution, and the Graduate School currently provides training for physicians in more than 85 specialties.

During its fledgling years, Mayo Graduate School of Medicine was under the direction of Dr. Louis B. Wilson (1915-1937). As its first director, Dr. Wilson played a key role in establishing the school and its programs. His successors, Drs. Donald C. Balfour (1937-1947) and Victor Johnson (1947-1966), continued to develop the graduate program through the austere years of World War II and the era of expansion that followed.

Subsequently, Mayo's educational commitments were broadened under the following Directors for Education: Drs. Charles F. Code (1966-1968), Raymond D. Pruitt (1968-1977), John T. Shepherd (1977-1983), and Franklyn G. Knox (1983 to date). Additional programs such as Mayo Medical School and Mayo School of Health-Related Sciences were instituted. This period of growth and development necessitated the appointment of several associate directors, and Mayo

284

Graduate School of Medicine currently has associate directors for each of the laboratory, medical, and surgical programs. Dr. Collin S. MacCarty was Director for Graduate Education from 1978 to 1980. The 1989 appointment of Dr. Alan D. Sessler as the first Dean of Mayo Graduate School of Medicine marked the beginning of another new era in the school's development.

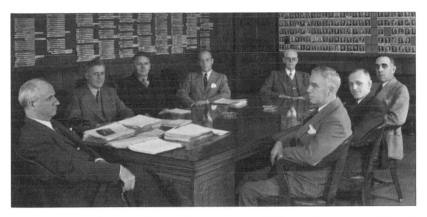

Members of the Graduate Committee of Mayo Graduate School of Medicine in 1941. Left, around the table: Drs. Donald C. Balfour, Sr. (director, 1937-1947), Russell M. Wilder, Frank C. Mann, James T. Priestley II, Louis B. Wilson (director, 1915-1937), Arlie R. Barnes, William F. Braasch, and Melvin S. Henderson. With establishment of the graduate school program in 1915, a graduate committee was formed to help with administration.

Mayo Alumni Association

Dr. Harold L. Foss led the Mayo Alumni Association in its beginning year, 1915. This group reflected the ideals instilled by the close association of its members with the Mayo brothers during those fledgling years.

The Mayo brothers frequently attended early meetings of the association. During the meeting in October 1919, the brothers reported on their establishment of Mayo Foundation. At this gathering, each brother also paid tribute to the new alumni organization.

In his remarks, Dr. Charlie, with his usual charming wit, noted: "Most of you are outwardly somewhat changed. We remember you when you worked in the operating rooms; then you weighed from 115 to 125 pounds; and it gives us the feeling that age is coming on to see you back here weighing from 160 to 200 pounds." He added that the success of the Clinic, in the future as well as in the past, was in no small measure due to the help of the alumni.

Dr. Will, in his more serious way, observed:

It is interesting to theorize on the possible influences that have contributed to the unusual growth of the Clinic. In view of the large number of sick who come here to be cared for, it would be natural to attribute the cause of their coming to work well done. But since good work is being done everywhere, there must be another and deeper reason.

Perhaps this other reason may best be summed up in one phrase, the spirit of the Clinic, into which is incorporated the desire to aid those who are suffering; the desire to advance in medical education by research, by diligent observation, and by the application of knowledge gained from others; and most important of all, the desire to pass on to others the scientific candle this spirit has lighted.

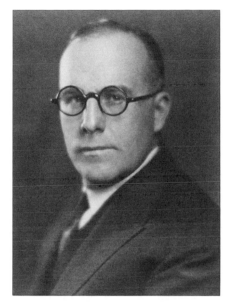

Dr. Harold L. Foss headed the newly formed Association of Resident and Ex-Resident Physicians of Mayo Clinic in 1915. Now called Mayo Alumni Association, its 10,000 members practice throughout the world.

Mayo Alumni Reunions

During the Mayo brothers' later years, a reunion of Mayo Graduate School alumni took place each year in Rochester. These gatherings usually included brief welcoming words from both of the brothers. At the 1930 meeting, Dr. William J. Mayo made a particularly revealing statement about the development of Mayo and its educational mission. In part, Dr. Will said:

When we began to practice, medicine was in a process of change and development. We had had the remarkable advantage of growing up with a pioneer surgeon and medical man of the old school, our father, and we not only had learned from him material facts but had gained an insight into the conditions which surrounded the sick and into the care necessary to them.

When we were boys, our mother used to say to Charlie and me, 'Don't think too much about the duties other people owe you, but rather about what your duty is to them . . .' As we grew older we realized more and more that success, in the best sense in which we use the word, often depends more on what we give than on what we receive.

One must remember always that when people are sick, they and their families will probably be more controlled by emotion than by intellect, and the art of the practice of medicine is to understand these emotions as well as to do the necessary material things for their welfare. So we traveled, one at a time, the world over, always striving to learn something which we could bring home and which would help us in our profession. In those days there was no place where one could go and learn more than a few things in medicine or surgery, because there was no center in which all things had been collected equally.

Away back in the '90s, my brother and I talked over these educational problems. We had no thought of being able to establish what might be called a clearinghouse in medicine, but we did hope that it might be possible to develop a group of men who could gather together medical knowledge, at least the most important facts, and pass them on to all who desired to learn . . .

Out of this tentative plan has grown the Clinic and the Foundation. Its value lies not in what our faithful colleagues and we have done, not in the material evidences of growth, but in the things of the spirit, the desire to develop a group of young men who would be more highly trained than ourselves, to take care of the sick. As the Clinic has grown, it has been the desire of us all to further not only investigations in pure science, but those humane investigations which will benefit the unfortunate who have undergone the trial of sickness, who started out in life with the same hopes, aspirations, and ambitions that we have, and too often through no fault of their own have been left by the wayside.

We have believed that the men who have been taught in the Clinic by our co-laborers as well as by ourselves would carry this concept of medicine to an increasing number of men and by their personal influence, induce them to do likewise; that thus, indefinitely as medicine progressed, would be maintained a group of scholars, teachers, gentlemen, who worked not for themselves but for the people whom they served. We must always remember that the hallmark of the gentleman is not his clothes or his manners, but his consideration for others.

I think, therefore, that you can see that the yearly return of the fellows who have worked with us and who show by their effort and their lives the same professional concept which we hold sacred is a source of pride, of satisfaction to us such as nothing else could give.

Saint Marys School of Nursing

Mabel Christensen and Matilda Kuethe became the first graduates of Saint Marys Training School in 1908. Sister Mary Joseph, Saint Marys' superintendent, had inaugurated the new nursing school in 1906. Anna Jamme, a graduate of Johns Hopkins School of Nursing, was the school's first head. Under her direction, the two-year diploma program quickly became a leader among the nursing schools of its day.

After Anna Jamme left in 1911, a series of short-term nursing superintendents followed: Anna Stone, Mary Meyer, and Elizabeth Lauer. After Mary C. Ledwidge was appointed superintendent in 1914, she initiated a three-year program at the school. Sisters M. Dionysia and M. Monica were the first Sisters to complete the new program in 1916.

Sister Mary Dionysia became school superintendent in 1920. She was followed by Mary Gladwin (1928), Sister M. Paul (1929), and Sister M. Domitilla (1932). When Sister M. Ancina took over the superintendent's post in 1934, her title changed to director of nurses. Sister M. Antonia (1937), Evalyne Collins (1947), and Sister M. Julie (1949) followed her as directors.

Over the years, the school's name evolved from Saint Marys Training School to Saint Marys Hospital School of Nursing (1932) and finally to Saint Marys School of Nursing (1949). The first men admitted to the school were Telmer Peterson and Emil Zahasky in 1937. Over the years, other alternatives in nursing education became available at Saint Marys through a baccalaureate program set up with the College of Saint Teresa in 1936 and the establishment of the Rochester School of Vocational Nursing in 1948.

The last class of Saint Marys School of Nursing graduated in June 1970. During the half-century of its existence, the school trained 3,830 graduates. Like the Methodist-Kahler School of Nursing, the Saint Marys school closed its doors in 1970.

Rochester Community College then became the major institution

290

in the city to offer an associate degree program in nursing. Sister Loretta Klinkhammer of Saint Marys became the associate director of this two-year program.

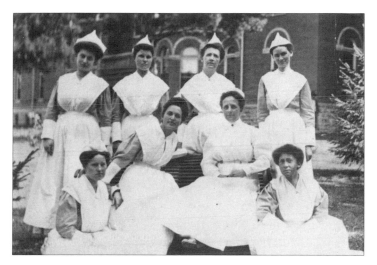

Sister Mary Joseph inaugurated Saint Marys Training School for nurses in 1906. This photograph shows students in the first two classes of the program with the school's head, Anna Jamme. Front row, left: Mary Shortner, Mabel Christensen, Superintendent Jamme, and Matilda Kuethe. Back row, left: Mona Van der Horck, Winnie Mertz, Elizabeth Stehm, and Sister William Fishenich. The school later became Saint Marys School of Nursing. (Courtesy Saint Marys Hospital.)

Methodist-Kahler School of Nursing

In 1918, the Colonial Hospital Training School for Nurses was established by the Kahler Corporation. Armed forces enlistments had caused a shortage of registered nurses locally, which affected the expanding Kahler hospital program. As a result, Dr. Melvin S. Henderson, chief of staff of Kahler's Colonial Hospital and Mayo's orthopedic head, and Mary J. Gill, R.N., Colonial superintendent of nurses, requested an emergency one-year training program.

Harriet M. Lisowski, R.N., was initially employed as the school's first instructor. In April 1918 the first five students enrolled. By fall, a total of 35 pupils had entered the new program; however, the end of the war during the next year caused a number of students to drop out of the school. Those who remained continued on in an expanded two-year program. The first 10 graduates of this program received their certificates and pins in 1920.

During that year, Mrs. Florence J. Wilson became Colonial superintendent and nursing head. Because of the press of her duties, it became necessary in the fall to employ Bertha S. Johnson as director of the nursing program. She soon launched an accredited three-year curriculum under the name of Colonial and Allied Hospitals' School of Nurses.

Twenty members of the school's original 1918 class completed the new three-year diploma program in 1921. During that year, the school's name changed to the Kahler Hospital's School of Nursing. A joint commencement was held in 1922 for the first graduates of 1921 and 1922.

The nursing program continued to grow and reached its peak enrollment of 473 in 1944, during World War II. When Methodist Hospital took over the Kahler Hospitals in 1954, the nursing school became known as the Methodist-Kahler School of Nursing. In 1970, the school issued its 3,827th diploma before closing. Rochester Community College then became the major institution granting nursing degrees in the city.

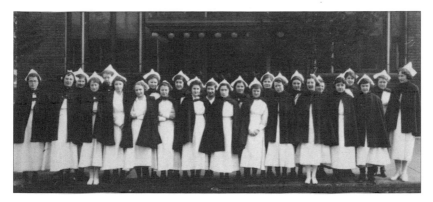

Colonial Hospital Training School for Nurses was established in 1918 by the Kahler Corporation. The Class of 1923 is pictured, shortly after the program became known as Kahler Hospital's School of Nursing, with a three-year diploma program. In 1954, Rochester Methodist Hospital took over the program and it became the Methodist-Kahler School of Nursing. (Courtesy Rochester Methodist Hospital.)

Physical Therapy School

The first physical therapy graduates at Mayo completed their training program, passed their registry examinations, and became senior registered physical therapy technicians in September 1939. The first class consisted of 14 members who began their training in Rochester on October 1, 1938.

The pioneering program came under the direction of Dr. Frank H. Krusen, its founder and head of the 16-member faculty. The program offered classes in light therapy, hydrotherapy, electrotherapy, occupational therapy, ethics, principles of apparatus, orthopedics, pathology, anatomy, physiology, neurology, chemistry, physics, bandaging, corrective exercise, massage, and kinesiology.

Carl E. Moe was named president of the graduating class. Members came from Minnesota, Wisconsin, and Canada. They published a yearbook called *Shortwave* and dedicated it to the Mayo brothers, who had died earlier that year.

Since those early days, the physical therapy program has grown at Mayo to become a 22-month course that offers a Master's degree in Physical Therapy.

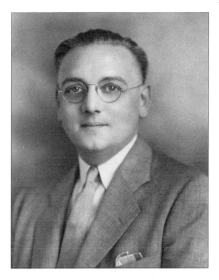

Dr. Frank H. Krusen arrived at Mayo in 1935 to start the Section on Physical Therapy (now Department of Physical Medicine and Rehabilitation). Dr. Krusen established Mayo Clinic School of Physical Therapy in 1938. The training program now offers a Master's degree in Physical Therapy.

Commencement Address by Dr. Will

The ritual of graduation from secondary and collegiate schools usually includes suitable words from some person of distinction. Over their careers, the Mayo brothers participated in a number of such ceremonies as commencement speakers. On June 15, 1910, Dr. William J. Mayo addressed graduates of Rush Medical College in Chicago. His remarks are sprinkled with suggestions that are timeless in their application. In part, Dr. Will said:

Your studies have not ended, but only just begun . . .

It is perhaps trite and commonplace to say—you must work. However, I believe that work and the manner of its accomplishment will make your success or your failure in the years to come.

Cultivate methodic habits of study. Remember that study is a part of your business and must be habitual and daily. I would suggest the plan of reading not less than one hour a day. If, when taking a vacation, or for any other cause you should lose some hours of study, keep a credit and debit ledger; a week means seven hours to make up. Never allow yourself to borrow from the future; not that you should confine yourself to one hour a day, but three or four hours' reading in one day should be not be used for credit in advance.

Take frequent vacations from active work, to attend clinics and walk hospital wards. See things for yourself; reading alone is not enough . . .

Write papers; they will do you much good, although at first they may not benefit any one else. In order to write papers you will institute a wider range of reading and investigation, you will learn to crystallize your thoughts and expressions, and finally, to produce work worthy of your efforts.

Attend your medical societies and take part in the discussions. The best man in your local society naturally takes a place in the district society; from the district to the state, and from the state to the national organizations.

I would admonish you, above all other considerations, to be honest. I mean honesty in every conception of the word: let it enter into all the details of your work; in the treatment of your patients and in your association with your brother practitioners. Should you have no stronger incentive, be assured that, to be other than fair, generous, and sincere, will ultimately spell ruin and not success . . .

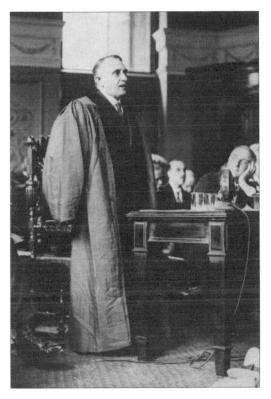

The Mayo brothers often participated in various educational programs. Here, Dr. Charlie speaks to the students of the London Hospital Medical College and Dental School.

Medical Editing at Mayo

On March 1, 1907, Maud H. Mellish Wilson came to Mayo Clinic "to organize and develop a library and to do editorial work in connection with the preparation of scientific publications." During the next 26 years, she became one of America's pioneer medical editors. In 1922, she prepared a small volume, *The Writing of Medical Papers*, which went through three editions and became a standard in the field of medical writing.

She was born Annie Maud Headline on February 14, 1862, near Faribault, Minnesota. Interested in medicine but having limited resources, she entered the training program for nurses at Presbyterian Hospital in Chicago, which had a close relationship with Rush Medical College. Enrolling at Presbyterian in 1885, she became the leading student in her nursing class. She also found time to attend medical school lectures at Rush. Even though she was not enrolled as a medical student, Dr. Moses Gunn and other members of the Rush faculty supported her efforts to acquire a medical education.

After graduation from nursing school in 1887, she became superintendent of the Maurice Porter Memorial Hospital for Children in Chicago. The responsibilities of the new position made it difficult for her to continue studying medicine. With her marriage to Dr. Ernest J. Mellish in 1889, she finally ended her pursuit of a medical degree.

Her marriage was immediately challenged by the effects of tuberculosis, which Dr. Mellish had previously contracted. Initially, the couple spent three years in northern Michigan, after which they returned to Chicago, where Dr. Mellish developed a fairly successful surgical practice. In 1901, they moved to Texas, and Dr. Mellish died there in 1905.

During the 16 years of this marriage, Mrs. Mellish dropped the name "Annie" at her husband's request and used "Maud." Besides the care of her ill spouse and handling their financial affairs, she helped edit her husband's scientific papers and those of Dr. A. J. Ochsner.

After her husband's death, Mrs. Mellish continued to assist Dr. Ochsner while undertaking the organization of a library for Augustana Hospital. During this period, Dr. William J. Mayo began looking for someone to assist editorially. On the basis of Dr. Ochsner's recommendation, Maud Mellish was invited to Mayo in

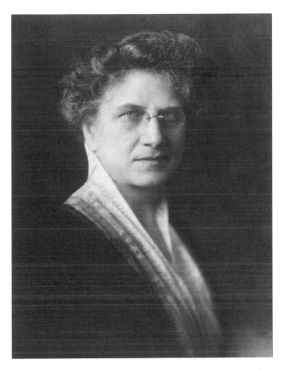

Maud Mellish Wilson joined Mayo in 1907 "to organize and develop a library and to do editorial work." She became one of America's pioneer medical editors. Before her death in 1933, she helped organize a rich medical library program and a pioneer medical graphics service, in addition to encouraging excellence in medical writing among her Mayo colleagues.

1907. Under her leadership, the editorial and library activities grew. In 1914, a Division of Publications was formed with an editorial section, a library, and an art studio. Mellish was named director of the new division and head of the editorial section. A trained librarian relieved her of the routine responsibilities of the library, and thereafter she devoted most of her time to editorial work.

In 1924, Mellish married Dr. Louis B. Wilson, who was then head of the Division of Laboratories at Mayo and director of Mayo Graduate School of Medicine. The marriage was a happy one, with both partners sharing an interest in each other's work.

During her Mayo career, Maud Mellish Wilson edited the *Collected Papers from the Mayo Clinic and the Mayo Foundation*, covering the period from 1905 to 1933. She inaugurated the weekly *Proceedings of the Staff Meetings of the Mayo Clinic* in 1926 (now *Mayo Clinic Proceedings*). She also handled the 11 volumes of the *Surgical Clinics of North America* and the 12 volumes of the *Medical Clinics of North America* that were contributed by Mayo authors during her career. Besides these works, she and her assistants processed eight Mayo Clinic monographs, four volumes of Mayo Foundation lectures, and the annual *Transactions of the Association of Resident and Ex-Resident Physicians of the Mayo Clinic and Mayo Foundation*. She and her associates also edited hundreds of medical papers that were written by the Mayo staff.

After an exploratory operation disclosed widespread abdominal cancer, Maud Mellish Wilson died on November 6, 1933. During her funeral services, Mayo Clinic closed. Dr. Will wrote a personal tribute that described her 26 years of educational work at Mayo as "the supreme monument to the life of a great lady."

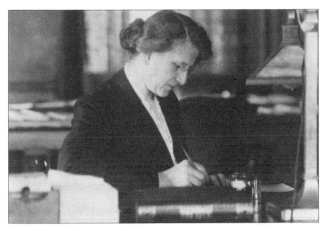

Maud Mellish Wilson at work in her office in the 1914 Mayo Clinic Building. As founder of the editorial activity, she was responsible for developing many Clinic publications.

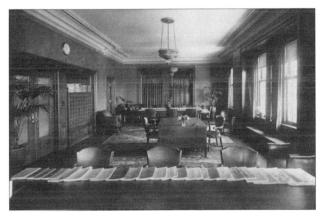

The main reading room of the Mayo medical library in the 1914 Clinic Building.

Maud H. Mellish Wilson Memorial Playground

Dr. Louis B. Wilson was Mayo's first pathologist and director of education, and his wife, Maud Mellish Wilson, was Mayo's first editor and librarian. The couple married in 1924, and together they developed a 50-acre tract of land into a productive farm homestead called Walnut Hill. Their farm, which adjoined Assisi Heights in northwest Rochester, included an orchard, a woodland area, several types of gardens, farm animals, and abundant wildlife.

The Wilsons hoped to share this beautiful setting with the children of Mayo families. After Mrs. Wilson's death in 1933, Dr. Wilson developed a unique outdoor program for children. He opened the Maud H. Mellish Wilson Memorial Playground in the summer of 1934. Its program, modeled after a similar plan at the University of Chicago, fostered social relationships among preschool-aged children. Initially, the program was limited to children of Mayo consultants and fellows, but it later expanded to include the three- to six-year-old children of all Mayo personnel. For more than a decade, Dr. Wilson and his new wife, Grace McCormick Wilson, continued the half-day playground on weekdays in June, July, and August.

Grace McCormick Wilson was the chief organizer and director of the program from its inception. She had been a close friend of Maud Mellish and was a child educator of several years' experience. Mothers of the children provided additional supervision.

After Dr. Wilson's death, Grace Wilson continued the program for several years with limited Mayo Foundation help. Because she was advancing in age and community education facilities were expanding, the project was discontinued in 1950.

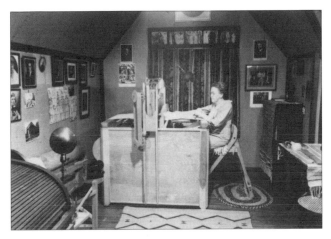

The marriage of Dr. Louis B. Wilson and Maud Mellish was a happy one. They shared their Walnut Hill home and its extensive grounds with other members of the Clinic family, particularly young children. Following Mrs. Wilson's death in 1933, Dr. Wilson established the Maud H. Mellish Wilson Memorial Playground at Walnut Hill in Northwest Rochester. Grace McCormick Wilson, shown at the loom, became director of the project, which continued for several years after Dr. Wilson's death in 1942.

The Wilsons and Walnut Hill

At the Clinic, Dr. Louis B. Wilson is commonly known as the first director of Mayo's education program and developer of the fresh frozen tissue method for pathological diagnosis in surgery. Knowledge of his avocational interest in horticulture surfaces only occasionally in local circles, with reference to Walnut Hill and the "potato king."

Born and raised in the farm lands of Pennsylvania, Dr. Wilson acquired a youthful interest in gardens and fruit trees that remained throughout his life. As he matured, he became a teacher of science and botany in midwestern secondary schools. When he arrived at Mayo as its first pathologist in 1905, he continued to pursue horticultural interests of some significance until his death in 1943.

In 1923, he purchased 41 acres on the bluffs then just north of the city limits. The tract later became part of the Assisi Heights grounds.

Dr. Wilson and his wife, Maud Mellish Wilson, named their new hilltop acreage Walnut Hill. They built a home there with interesting features designed by Harold H. Crawford. Around its grounds flourished a variety of gardens. To the north, Dr. Wilson planted his first orchard in 1925. It had alternating rows of apple and plum trees of the latest Minnesota varieties. The Haralson apple became Dr. Wilson's favorite and on a good year, it accounted for some 3,200 bushels of the orchard's total production of 5,000 bushels.

In this orchard, Dr. Wilson grew Green Mountain potatoes between the tree rows. Their yield was so great that the finest were sold to midwestern railroads. As a result, Dr. Wilson became locally known as the "potato king."

During the late 1920s, Dr. Bastianelli of Rome, physician to the Italian monarchy, visited Mayo. Dr. and Mrs. Wilson hosted him at Walnut Hill. He savored the Wilson's homegrown potatoes.

When Dr. Wilson visited Premier Mussolini in 1926, along with other medical dignitaries, Dr. Bastianelli introduced him as a most knowledgeable man on potatoes. The Italian farmers needed increased productivity at this time. As a result of the Wilson interview, an Italian potato commission was later appointed, and members visited America to study its methods.

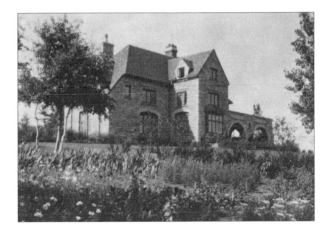

The Walnut Hill farm of Dr. L. B. Wilson and his wife, Maud, featured an orchard that alternated rows of apple and plum trees. The Haralson apple was Dr. Wilson's favorite and its trees yielded some 3,200 bushels on a good year. Between the tree rows, Green Mountain potatoes were grown and often sold to the railroads, giving Dr. Wilson the local title of "potato king."

The Wilson Club

On December 13, 1934, the Association of Fellows held a meeting in Rochester under the leadership of its president, Dr. Harrison R. Wesson. The proceedings noted that the Club's new quarters were nearly completed and that a name should be chosen.

After discussion, the group decided the name should honor a living individual. Among those proposed, Dr. John McGowan suggested Wilson Club, honoring Dr. Louis B. Wilson, first director of Mayo Graduate School of Medicine. A vote was taken, and Wilson Club became the new facility's name.

An announcement of the club's opening appeared in the *Clinic Bulletin* on December 29, 1934. According to a news note, an open house took place that same day between 3 and 5 p.m.

The Wilson Club was located at 212 Second Street, Southwest, on the site of the present Hilton Building. The building was erected around 1913 by Archie P. Gove and Elmer E. Howe as the Waukesha Hotel. Shortly thereafter, it became the Laurence Hotel and remained so until Mayo purchased the structure around 1933.

After the building was remodeled and reopened as the Wilson Club, the three-story structure became a popular gathering place for Mayo residents. The rooms upstairs provided quarters for about a dozen bachelor residents. On the lower floors, the club featured a dining room that served breakfast and lunch, a library, game rooms, a darkroom, and lounge areas.

With the opening of the Harwick cafeteria in 1966, the Wilson Club's dining room service was discontinued. The Wilson Club itself was finally closed on September 1, 1970, and subsequently razed to make way for the Hilton Building.

During the 1970s and '80s, the Harwick Building contained a faculty dining hall known as the Wilson Room. With the opening of the Siebens Building, this facility moved to new quarters.

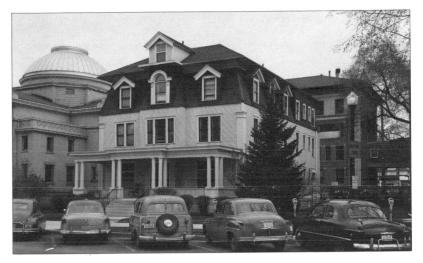

The Wilson Club was opened to the residents of Mayo Graduate School of Medicine in December 1934. Located on the site of the Hilton Building, the facility was formerly the Laurence Hotel. The club was popular with unmarried residents at Mayo. A dining room served breakfast and lunch, and rooms were available for single residents. Construction of the Hilton Building in the 1970s caused the Club to close.

Mayo Staff Trained in Canada

Over the years, Canadian universities have provided Mayo with a number of staff members who have made significant contributions to the development of its programs. In 1964, a tabulation indicated that from eight to 10 percent of the Mayo Graduate School of Medicine residents came from Canadian schools each year. By the time the Mayo brothers died in 1939, some 28 Canadian-trained physicians had entered Mayo and been appointed consultants or would be appointed consultants later.

Dr. Melvin S. Henderson was the first to arrive with Canadian academic credentials. He was a St. Paul, Minnesota, native who had lived in Canada since the age of seven. After completing medical school and an internship, Dr. Henderson entered the Clinic as a surgical assistant in June 1907. After assisting the Mayo brothers in surgery, he founded Mayo's Section on Orthopaedic Surgery in 1912. While heading this pioneering section, he also served as a member and officer of Mayo's governing boards. Dr. Henderson retired in 1950 and died in 1954.

Shortly after Dr. Henderson's arrival in Rochester, he notified Dr. Donald C. Balfour, his medical school friend, of an opening in pathology at the Clinic. Dr. Balfour took the next train to Rochester from Canada and won the assistantship in pathology on July 7, 1907. Later he transferred his interest to surgery and became head of a section on general surgery in 1912. He also became a member of the Mayo partnership and helped establish the graduate school program and Mayo Properties Association (today's Mayo Foundation). Dr. Balfour was chief of the division of surgery from 1923 to 1935 and director of Mayo Graduate School of Medicine from 1937 to 1947. He retired in 1947 and died in 1963.

Besides these two early Mayo associates, the following Mayo consultants with Canadian university degrees entered the Clinic during the Mayo brothers' era:

Gordon B. New (1910-1949)

Harry G. Wood (1911-1916, 1926-1947)

James C. Masson (1912-1949)

Russell D. Carman (1913-1918)

Willis S. Lemon (1917-1946)

Charles G. Sutherland (1918-1942)

Leonard G. Rowntree (1920-1932)

Norman M. Keith (1920-1950)

James F. Weir (1920-1958)

D. Morrison Masson (1921-1957)

Charles S. McVicar 1921-1929)

W. Berkeley Stark (1922-1934)

Edward J. Baldes (1924-1963)

Frank N. Allan (1925-1932)

Haddow M. Keith (1928-1932, 1939-1964)

Ralph M. Tovell (1929-1936)

John R. McDonald (1933-1958)

Charles F. Code (1934-1975)

Malcolm B. Dockerty (1934-1974)

Carl G. Morlock (1934-1975)

Alexander R. MacLean (1934-1952)

R. Charles Adams (1935-1956)

Thomas H. Seldon (1936-1970)

Howard B. Burchell (1936-1967)

Deward O. Ferris (1937-1972)

Allan A. Bailey (1937-1940, 1947-1954)

George P. Sayre (1939-1975)

Joseph M. Janes (1939-1974).

· SECTION VIII ·

Mayo Accomplishments and Activities

Over the years, Mayo people have engaged in a wide range of activities that resulted in scientific contributions of lasting importance. The Mayo brothers encouraged and supported individual achievement. Their interest in the development of new knowledge stimulated their colleagues to reach beyond the known.

Thyroxine Isolated

Early in this century, Dr. Edward C. Kendall completed at Mayo the final steps in the isolation of thyroxine, the hormone of the thyroid gland. While working in the biochemical laboratory in the 1914 Mayo Clinic Building during the evening of December 23, 1914, Dr. Kendall dissolved and separated the acid-soluble fraction that he had spent some three years isolating.

Up to that point, he had only been able to separate a compound that contained 47 percent iodine. By using ethanol as a solvent that December evening, he was able to dissolve a sample of the fraction. While waiting for the alcohol to dissipate and leave a more concentrated solution, he fell asleep. Upon awakening, Dr. Kendall saw that all the alcohol had disappeared and a white crust remained, surrounded by a ring of yellowish, waxy material. He found that alcohol would dissolve the waxy substance and leave the white crust intact.

The next morning, an analysis of the white material showed that it contained 60 percent iodine. Further tests were made. On Christmas morning, the white crust was dissolved using ethanol that contained sodium hydroxide. A few drops of acetic acid then precipitated the material into a fine crystalline form, and Dr. Kendall's search was over. Thyroxine, as he later named it, had been isolated.

Afterward, Mayo Staff spent several years developing the adequate means for producing the hormone in quantity and determining its structure and properties. Chemical analysis showed that the hormone was composed of the following percentages of: carbon (22.37), hydrogen (1.65), oxygen (8.73), nitrogen (2.23), and iodine (65.02). Dr. Kendall summarized the research in a definitive publication in 1918. In the meantime, treatment of patients with the thyroid gland hormone often produced dramatic, satisfying results. Later, Dr. C. R. Harington, working in London, finally synthesized the compound in 1926, and Dr. Kendall prepared a monograph on the subject in 1928.

The isolation of thyroxine was but the first of a series of accomplishments by Dr. Kendall and his laboratory associates. His work culminated in 1950 when he and Dr. Philip S. Hench received the Nobel Prize for their work in developing cortisone.

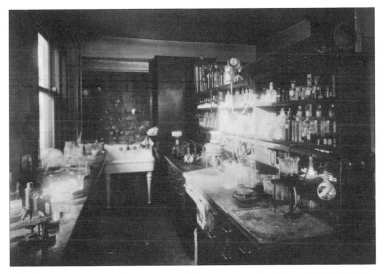

In this first biochemistry laboratory in the 1914 Clinic Building, Dr. Edward C. Kendall isolated thyroxine, hormone of the thyroid gland, on December 23, 1914. Working in the evening, Dr. Kendall fell asleep, and awoke to find his solution had precipitated into a compound that finally yielded 60 percent iodine. The new hormone often produced dramatic, beneficial results in patients.

Basal Metabolic Rate Determination

Early in 1917, Dr. Walter M. Boothby and his first assistant, Irene Sandiford, arrived at Mayo from Boston. They had been appointed in November 1916 to develop a laboratory of basal metabolism at the Clinic. Between 1913 and 1916, Dr. Boothby had been in charge of the metabolism laboratory at Peter Bent Brigham Hospital. At Mayo, they initially focused their studies on the metabolism of patients with hypothyroidism and hyperthyroidism.

Shortly after his arrival, Dr. Boothby left the Clinic for military service. During his absence, Irene Sandiford conducted the laboratory work under the supervision of Dr. Henry S. Plummer.

About the time Dr. Boothby returned from the service in 1919, Sandiford received her Ph.D. degree from the University of Minnesota. Until Dr. Sandiford left the Clinic in 1930 for the University of Chicago, she and Dr. Boothby collaborated in studies that developed reliable laboratory procedures for determining basal metabolic rate. In 1920, they published a fundamental work, *Laboratory Manual of a Technic of Basal Metabolic Rate Determinations.*

Until his retirement from Mayo in 1948, Dr. Boothby maintained an interest in this subject. Among his 300 scientific papers, the field of metabolism is prominent, along with respiration, thyroid disease, and aviation medicine.

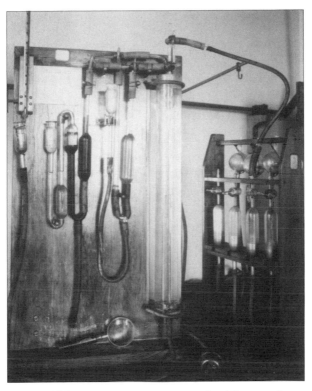

The Haldane Analyzer was a significant piece of equipment used by Drs. Walter M. Boothby and Irene Sandiford in developing their technique for determining basal metabolic rate. Their findings were published in a classic laboratory manual in 1920.

Vitamin C and Mayo

In 1937, Dr. Albert Szent-Gyorgyi von Nagyrapolt received the Nobel Prize in Physiology and Medicine. The award recognized his discoveries in the biological combustion processes with special reference to vitamin C. Interestingly, between 1929 and 1930, Dr. Szent-Gyorgyi used the facilities of Dr. E. C. Kendall's laboratory at Mayo for some of his basic work with the new compound.

Before coming to Rochester, Dr. Szent-Gyorgyi isolated several small amounts of the compound that were widely distributed in fruits, vegetables, and animals. He named his discovery "hexuronic acid." The highest concentration of the substances was then found in the adrenal glands. Working in England, Dr. Szent-Gyorgyi was hindered by a limited supply of the glands.

Aware of Dr. Kendall's work at Mayo, Dr. Szent-Gyorgyi requested permission to become a visiting scientist in Kendall's laboratory. He hoped to use bovine adrenal glands from St. Paul packing houses to complete his isolation work of hexuronic acid. His request was approved, and Szent-Gyorgyi and his wife arrived in Rochester in the fall of 1929. They were an outgoing couple and soon developed many friends locally.

When they left Rochester in May 1930, Dr. Szent-Gyorgyi had isolated several more grams of hexuronic acid. Some initially negative reports about its relationship with vitamin C had discouraged him, however, from undertaking further physiologic studies of the compound. Several years later, he continued his investigation and established that hexuronic acid and vitamin C were the same compound. He received the Nobel Prize shortly thereafter.

After Szent-Gyorgyi left Rochester, Kendall and his clinical associates became interested in the hormones of the adrenal cortex. The wooden press, large meat grinder, and 40-gallon crocks left from Szent-Gyorgyi's studies enabled Kendall to begin the chemical investigation of the adrenal cortex, which culminated in Drs. Kendall and Hench receiving the Nobel Prize in 1950.

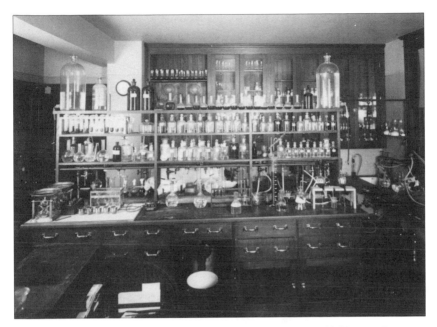

The Kendall laboratory in the 1914 Clinic Building. Szent-Gyorgyi utilized these facilities to continue his studies in hexuronic acid. For some nine months, he and his wife were in Rochester while he refined a few grams of the compound. Tests by an interested colleague abroad failed to establish a connection with vitamin C. Szent-Gyorgyi left Rochester discouraged and did not complete his studies until some years later. He received the Nobel Prize for the work's completion.

Cancer Grading System or Broders' Index

In 1920, Dr. Albert C. Broders of Mayo's pathology staff published the first of four papers describing a system of microscopically grading cancers on a numerical basis, with 1 denoting a cancer of the least malignancy and 4 the highest malignancy.

Appearing in the *Journal of the American Medical Association*, Dr. Broders' paper, "Squamous-Cell Epithelioma of the Lip: A Study of 537 Cases," provided the beginnings of an index of malignancy that hospitals all over the world have adopted, thus bringing international recognition to its author and Mayo.

Albert Compton Broders was born on August 8, 1885. He was a native of Virginia and received most of his education there. Dr. Broders came to the Clinic in 1912 as an assistant in surgical pathology. He became an associate in pathology in 1919 and head of Section B in Surgical Pathology in 1922.

In addition to his cancer classification publications, Dr. Broders prepared another classic pathology paper, "Carcinoma 'In Situ' Contrasted With Benign Penetrating Epithelium," for the *Journal of the American Medical Association* in 1932. He also modified, in 1931, Dr. Louis B. Wilson's fresh frozen tissue technique that was originally developed for surgical use at Mayo in 1905.

Dr. Broders was director of the Division of Surgical Pathology at the Clinic from 1945 until his retirement in 1950. Afterwards, he joined the Scott and White Clinic and remained active in Texas until his death on March 27, 1964.

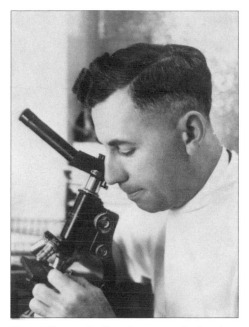

Dr. Albert C. Broders, pathologist, developed an index of malignancy at Mayo in 1920. His microscopic grading system was adopted by hospitals around the world. Dr. Broders entered Mayo in 1912 and retired in 1950.

Flour Enrichment

In 1938, at a meeting of the Council on Foods and Nutrition of the American Medical Association, Mayo's Dr. Russell M. Wilder proposed that the American milling industry add thiamine to white flour. The council agreed, and in early 1939 announced their initial recommendations for flour enrichment. Their statement helped stimulate General Mills, Inc., to produce a white flour with some of its micronutrients restored.

The movement to improve the nutritional quality of white flour had been growing since 1870, when a new roller milling process was introduced in America. While the new process produced a more appealing and better-textured flour, it caused health concerns among physicians and nutritionists because it removed nutritional elements from the wheat grain. The milling industry also had some concerns, but it feared that a return to the rough, gray flour of the past would diminish consumer appeal.

As the consumer-manufacturer dialogue developed, one proposal was to fortify white flour with the elements lost in milling. The synthesis of thiamine helped stimulate interest in this approach. Dr. Wilder recognized from his metabolic and nutrition work at Mayo what benefits such a program would bring. He became a prominent supporter of white flour enrichment and, as a result, was appointed the first chairman of the Food and Nutrition Board of the National Research Council in 1940. The new group played a key role in developing nutritional standards for white flour.

To help define which nutrients humans need that were removed from flour, Dr. Wilder enlisted the support of other Mayo colleagues such as Drs. G. M. Higgins, H. L. Mason, M. H. Power, B. F. Smith, and R. D. Williams in conducting a series of experimental studies between 1939 and 1942 on thiamine deficiency and human requirements, along with those of riboflavin. These studies, and others, helped the national bureaucracy to issue orders between 1941 and 1943 that covered levels for the enrichment of flour and bread with thiamine, riboflavin, niacin, iron, calcium, and Vitamin D.

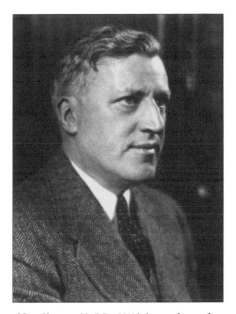

Dr. Russell M. Wilder played a key role in developing nutritional standards for white flour in the 1940s. He promoted white flour enrichment. Wilder was the first chairman of the Food and Nutrition Board of the National Research Council.

BLB Oxygen Mask

Shortly before the start of World War II, three Mayo investigators announced the development of a new type of oxygen inhalation mask for use in clinical medicine and high-altitude aviation. In the October 12, 1938, issue of the *Proceedings of the Staff Meetings of the Mayo Clinic*, Drs. Walter M. Boothby, W. Randolph Lovelace II, and Arthur H. Bulbulian first reported research and observations that led to the perfection of the apparatus. The new mask was dubbed the BLB oxygen mask after the names of its three designers.

The mask initially developed as part of Mayo's response to an inquiry from Northwest Airlines. Aviation was then on the brink of a new era in which aviators and passengers would routinely fly at altitudes above 12,000 feet (3,658 m). The potential risks of oxygen deficiency at higher elevations were unknown. Mayo investigators used the new mask and its specially developed oxygen supply equipment to determine oxygen requirements of human volunteers in a laboratory environment that simulated various altitudes.

To ensure controlled atmospheric conditions, Mayo installed, in 1939, the first low-pressure chamber in a civilian laboratory in the United States. Dr. Lovelace was assigned to the new facility full-time; along with his chief (Dr. Boothby) and some technicians, he proceeded to investigate the unknowns of high-altitude physiology.

These investigations had their roots in studies of anoxia conducted by Dr. Boothby since 1918 in Mayo's metabolism laboratory. In 1925, special chambers were installed to study oxygen therapy. Between 1938 and 1939, Dr. Boothby and his associates used these chambers in the developmental phases of the BLB mask by adding nitrogen to help simulate height.

As their high-altitude studies progressed, Drs. Boothby and Lovelace conducted several tests on long-distance flights in airplanes supplied by Northwest Airlines and fitted with Mayo masks and oxygen equipment. The success of these flights demonstrated the efficacy of providing oxygen during regular passenger service at high altitudes. In 1940, President Roosevelt honored the Mayo investigations when he presented the Collier Trophy, the highest aviation award in the United States, to Mayo's Boothby and Lovelace, along with Capt. Harry G. Armstrong of the U.S. Army, for their efforts in promoting aviation safety with a special emphasis on preventing pilot fatigue.

These events and the experimental data compiled by the Mayo investigative team, which included a practical method for

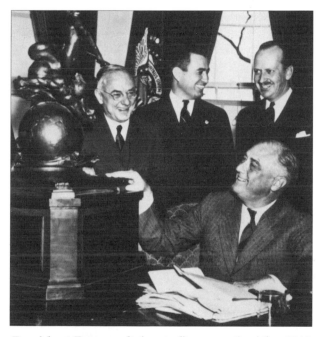

President Roosevelt (seated) presenting the 1940 Collier Trophy to Drs. Walter B. Boothby (left) and W. Randolph Lovelace, along with Capt. Harry Anderson. The highest U.S. aviation award, the trophy was given for the promotion of aviation safety, which included the work of Boothby and Lovelace with the BLB oxygen mask.

preventing decompression sickness (bends) in pilots, further stimulated national interest. As a result, pilots, aircraft designers, and military leaders came to Rochester to learn, and often participated in the studies.

In the early 1940s, Mayo Foundation organized a special Mayo Aero Medical Unit to further the aviation medicine work. Its facilities enlarged in 1942 with the addition of an acceleration laboratory, including a Mayo-designed human centrifuge. With the advent of World War II, the two laboratories of the Mayo Aero Medical Unit were made available to the U.S. Government at no expense as part of Mayo's assistance in the war effort. During this period, the Mayo team modified the BLB mask and its oxygen

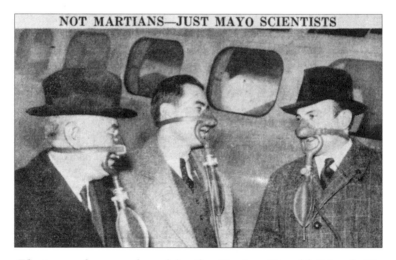

Photograph reproduced in the *Boston Herald*, March 11, 1939, upon arrival of Mayo researchers and their party after a four and one-half hour flight from Minneapolis, Minnesota, at speeds exceeding 250 miles per hour and elevations reaching 23,000 feet. Wearing the original BLB mask are Drs. W. W. Boothby (left), W. R. Lovelace and A. H. Bulbulian.

equipment many times to meet the special needs of the military. One of these modifications had a production run of more than a million units. In the decades that followed the war, the BLB oxygen mask was the prototype for all subsequently developed oxygen masks.

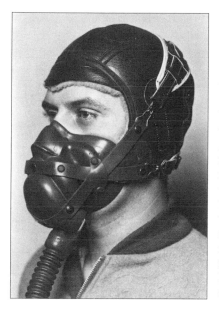

Fearing poison-gas attacks from Germany and learning of the Mayo mask, British scientists visited the Clinic to learn about oxygen therapy. During World War II, Mayo investigators also worked closely with the U.S. Army and Navy to improve the mask and oxygen equipment for military aircraft. The BLB team finally developed this A-14 "demand system" mask, which automatically controlled oxygen supply and allowed flights up to 38,000 feet. Mayo made this mask available to British and American units during the conflict.

Lindbergh at Mayo

During World War II, Charles A. Lindbergh was among the distinguished scientists, aviators, and other military personnel who visited Mayo's Aero Medical Unit. In the fall of 1942, Lindbergh and Dr. Charles J. Clark came to Rochester from the Ford Motor Company's Willow Run Bomber Plant for indoctrination in the Clinic's low-pressure chamber. During the visit, September 22 to October 3, Lindbergh made several simulated parachute jumps in the chamber from 40,000-foot altitudes. As a result of these experiments, Lindbergh and Dr. Walter M. Boothby, the unit's chairman, prepared two memorandum reports, "Observations, Experiences, and Recommendations Related to Bailing Out at High Altitudes," and "Report on Positive Pressure Breathing (A) Constant (B) Pulsating." After his return to Michigan, Lindbergh used the information from Rochester in his work with Ford Motor's new P-47 pursuit planes.

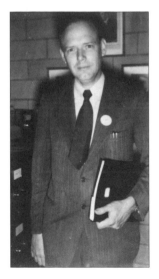

Charles A. Lindbergh visited Rochester in 1942 to use the resources of Mayo's Aero Medical Unit.

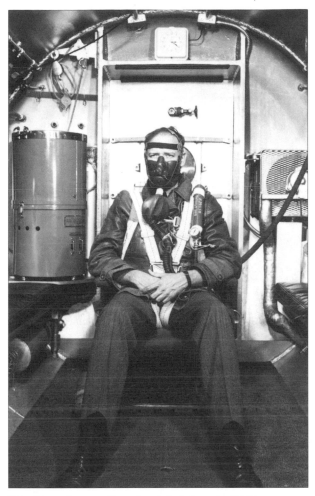

Lindbergh, outfitted with Mayo's BLB oxygen mask, tested bail-out techniques for the P-47 pursuit aircraft.

Mayo in the Pacific

It was in 1940 that the 71st Army General Hospital was organized in Rochester as a preparedness measure, since American involvement in World War II appeared possible. Many of the hospital's officers and allied personnel were recruited from the Clinic and Rochester.

In January 1943, the hospital was activated in Charleston, South Carolina. On June 24, 1943, its personnel were assigned to either the 233rd or 237th Station Hospitals. The new detachments received additional training in Charleston, and in the case of the 237th, a short period in Utica, New York.

In January 1944, both units were sent from Camp Stoneman, California, to New Guinea. The 233rd erected a station hospital there at Nadzab and the 237th built one at Finschhafen.

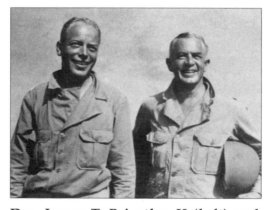

Drs. James T. Priestley II (left) and Charles W. Mayo commanded the two Mayo Army hospital units that served in the South Pacific during World War II. The units were derived from the 71st General Hospital organized in Rochester in 1940. Following service in New Guinea and the Phillipines, the hospitals were deactivated and their personnel returned to the United States.

On October 15, 1944, the 233rd Station Hospital, with expanded facilities, was redesignated the 247th General Hospital. Along with the 237th Station Hospital, it continued to care for patients in New Guinea until the middle of 1945.

In that year, both units were individually moved to the Philippines. The 247th was set up near Clark Field, and the 237th at Batangas. Both units served at these locations for the remainder of the war. Later, the Surgeon General of the United States Army issued certificates of appreciation to the Clinic in recognition of contributions these hospitals made to the war effort.

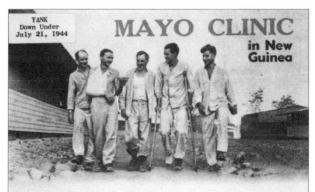

The Army publication *Yank Down Under* reported on Mayo's hospital units.

Nobel Prize in Physiology and Medicine

On December 10, 1950, Drs. Edward C. Kendall and Philip S. Hench of Mayo and Professor Tadeus Reichstein of Switzerland received the Nobel Prize in Physiology and Medicine for their "discoveries regarding the hormones of the adrenal cortex, their structure and biological effects."

The Nobel presentations took place in Stockholm, Sweden. King Gustave VI, the recently installed king of Sweden, presented each man with the Nobel Prize and citation. The ceremonies were particularly impressive since the Nobel Foundation was celebrating its 50th anniversary, and 26 Nobel laureates were in attendance.

Besides physiology and medicine, the awards in physics, chemistry, and literature were also presented on that occasion. Along with William Faulkner, who won the Nobel Prize in Literature, Drs. Kendall and Hench were the only American recipients in that ceremony. Ralph J. Bunche, another American, received the Nobel Peace Prize at a separate event.

On December 11, the Nobel Prize winners for 1950 gave lectures describing the work for which they were being honored. Dr. Hench, who earned the M.D. degree at the University of Pittsburgh, spoke on "The Reversibility of Certain Rheumatic and Non-Rheumatic Conditions by the Use of Cortisone or of the Pituitary Adrenocorticotropic Hormone." Dr. Kendall, who received his Ph.D. from Columbia University, spoke on "The Development of Cortisone as a Therapeutic Agent."

In these presentations, the Mayo authors reviewed their laboratory and clinical work, which spanned two decades. Dr. Kendall and his associates had started the tedious task of separating 28 different compounds from the adrenal cortex in the early 1930s. When compound E, or cortisone, became available in 1948, Drs. Hench and Kendall and their associates initiated the clinical trials that culminated in the announcement of their encouraging preliminary results in April 1949. The publication of their data brought them international recognition and finally the Nobel Prize.

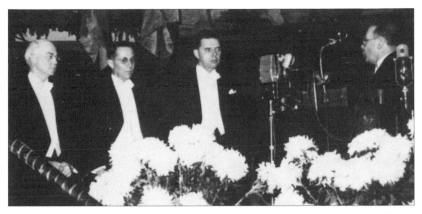

Drs. Edward C. Kendall (left), Philip S. Hench and Tadeus Reichstein received the Nobel Prize in Physiology and Medicine in Stockholm, Sweden, on December 10, 1950.

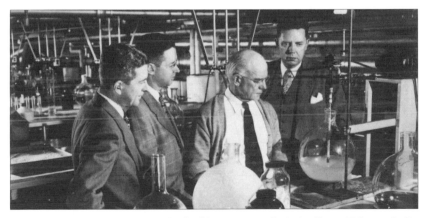

Drs. Charles H. Slocumb (left), Howard F. Polley, Edward C. Kendall and Philip S. Hench gathered in Kendall's biochemistry laboratory in 1949. Kendall and his laboratory colleagues, Drs. Harold L. Mason, Bernard McKenzie and Vernon R. Mattox, began the tedious chemical analysis of 28 hormones of the adrenal glands in the early 1930s. Dr. Hench and his clinical colleagues, Drs. Charles H. Slocumb and Howard F. Polley, initiated the clinical trials of cortisone in 1948.

Pioneering Chemotherapy Research

On January 29, 1945, Drs. William H. Feldman and H. Corwin Hinshaw completed their 166-day treatment of guinea pigs inoculated with virulent tubercle bacilli. Using recently discovered streptomycin, Feldman and Hinshaw demonstrated the "unquestionable ability of streptomycin to reverse the potentially lethal course of well-established inoculation tuberculosis in guinea pigs, and the relatively low toxicity and corresponding safety of purified streptomycin."

After this pioneering experiment at Mayo, Drs. Feldman and Hinshaw began almost immediately their equally successful study of treating tuberculosis among people with streptomycin at the Mineral Springs Sanatorium in Cannon Falls, Minnesota. Dr. Karl H. Pfuetze, medical superintendent at Mineral Springs, collaborated.

During their research, Drs. Feldman and Hinshaw were composed and consistent in handling the news media reports. They made every effort to prevent the public and the medical profession from becoming overly optimistic about their results. They pointed out that the drug did not provide a fast cure, but did alter the course of tuberculosis in a favorable manner and did suppress progressive types of the disease.

Drs. Feldman and Hinshaw are credited with establishing the "first disciplined scientific laboratory principles of chemotherapy evaluation."

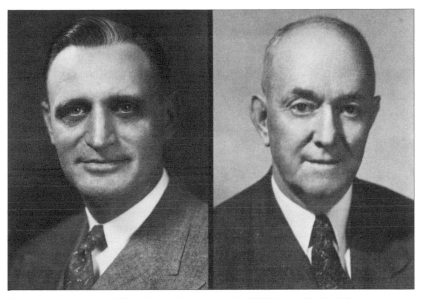

Drs. H. Corwin Hinshaw (left) and William H. Feldman were pioneer investigators in the treatment of tuberculosis with streptomycin in 1945. A doctor of veterinary medicine, Feldman had studied the disease since 1920. Dr. Hinshaw joined this fundamental work in chemotherapy in the 1930s.

Open-Heart Surgery at Mayo

The first heart-lung bypass operation in Rochester was done by Dr. John W. Kirklin on March 22, 1955. Working in the Colonial Building of Rochester Methodist Hospital, Dr. Kirklin's surgical team successfully corrected a ventricular septal defect on a five-year-old girl.

The operation ushered in the era of open-heart surgery at Mayo. It was the outgrowth of several years' planning by Drs. Kirklin and Earl H. Wood. Mayo's Section of Engineering, headed by Richard E. Jones, built a modified version of Dr. John H. Gibbon's mechanical pump-oxygenator. This specialized equipment allowed surgeons a "dry field" while operating on the heart.

During this period, there were different types of bypass devices. A mechanical pump-oxygenator system had worked successfully on two heart operations before Mayo began its work. Dr. J. H. Gibbon in Philadelphia and Dr. Clarence Crafoord in Sweden had been individually successful using such a device.

Prominent among those who helped develop Mayo's specifications for the bypass machine were Drs. David E. Donald, H. J. C. Swan, Harry G. Harshbarger, John W. Kirklin, and Earl H. Wood. Experimental laboratory work, conducted before the machine was used on humans, was carried out by Drs. Peter S. Hetzel and Robert T. Patrick, along with Drs. Kirklin, Wood, Donald, and Harshbarger. Also cooperating was Dr. J. H. Grindlay, assisted by non-medical personnel in surgical research.

The dramatic operation was a typical Mayo team effort that crossed many specialty areas. Prominent among the paramedical contributors was James Fellows, who assisted in operating the bypass device. Other technical assistants on the project included Lucille Cronin, Betty Hennessey, Owen Ellingson, Fred Williams, and William Sutterer. Surgical nurses included Delores Miller, Shirley Reusser, and Elizabeth Goodwyne.

334

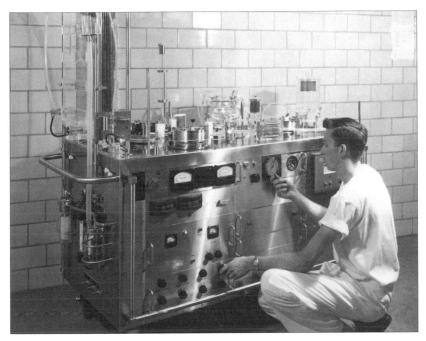

On March 22, 1955, the first heart-lung bypass operation in Rochester was performed by Dr. John W. Kirklin and his surgical team in the Colonial Building of Rochester Methodist Hospital. Using this version of the bypass machine, surgeons corrected a ventricular septal defect in a five-year-old girl. Mayo's Engineering Section designed and built the pioneering machine, which modified designs produced elsewhere.

Mayo Centennial

In 1964, a year-long celebration honored the Mayo Centennial. Beginning in January, a variety of special events took place in Rochester, including 42 scientific meetings and 20 programs that often involved community participation.

This Mayo Centennial Year commemorated the births of the Mayo brothers a century earlier and the 50th anniversary of the Mayo Graduate School of Medicine. Dr. Will was born in 1861 and Dr. Charlie in 1865. The year 1964 was a suitable time between their births in which to honor them.

A Mayo Centennial Committee was appointed by the Board of Governors to plan the complex undertaking. Dr. C. S. MacCarty headed the group as chairman. One of their first tasks was to commission an attractive seal that was designed by Gerald Hazzard. It became the symbol of the year and was cast in a limited edition as a souvenir.

The main activities of the year occurred in the fall. On September 11, 1964, dedication ceremonies for the United States commemorative Mayo postage stamp took place in Rochester with U.S. Postmaster General John A. Gronouski as the principal speaker. The Rochester Philatelic Club designed the official cachet, with the "First Day of Issue" from the Rochester Post Office.

September 16, 17, and 18, 1964, featured the Mayo Centennial Symposium. The Minneapolis Symphony Orchestra, conducted by Stanislaw Skrowaczewski, gave a special concert to begin the two-day international symposium.

Entitled Mirror to Man, the symposium's theme was "Man's Adaption to His Expanding Environment." Dr. L. M. Gould served as moderator for a distinguished panel of speakers that included Drs. C. A. Doxiadis, Loren Eiseley, Arthur Larson, Peter Brian Medawar, Edward Teller, and General Lauris Norstad.

During the symposium, the Mayo Centennial Convocation took place on September 17, 1964, with Dr. O. Meridith Wilson, president of the University of Minnesota, officiating. During the program, 35 outstanding achievement awards were given to former Mayo Foundation fellows.

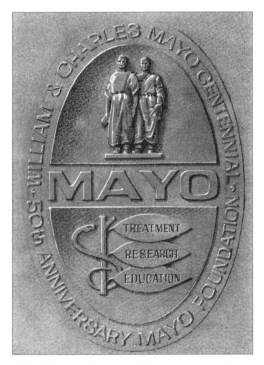

The Mayo Centennial was a year-long celebration during 1964. It honored the 100th anniversary of the Mayo brothers' births and the 50th anniversary of Mayo Graduate School. A special seal was commissioned by the Mayo Centennial Committee. Gerald Hazzard designed the symbol, which was used on publications and cast as a souvenir of the year's events.

· LISTING OF NAMES ·

Here are names of individuals who appear in the text and illustrations of this book. For information about Dr. William Worrall Mayo and his sons, Dr. William James Mayo and Dr. Charles Horace Mayo, please consult the Table of Contents.